Comprehensive review for

MEDICAL TECHNOLOGISTS

MOSBY'S COMPREHENSIVE REVIEW SERIES

Comprehensive review for
MEDICAL TECHNOLOGISTS

Edited by

ALICE M. SEMRAD

Director of Medical Technology,
Marquette University,
Milwaukee, Wisconsin

SECOND EDITION

THE C. V. MOSBY COMPANY

ST. LOUIS • TORONTO • LONDON   1979

SECOND EDITION

Copyright © 1979 by The C. V. Mosby Company

Previous edition copyrighted 1975

Printed in the United States of America

The C. V. Mosby Company
11830 Westline Industrial Drive, St. Louis, Missouri 63141

Library of Congress Cataloging in Publication Data

Semrad, Alice M   1929-
  Comprehensive review for medical technologists.

  (Mosby's comprehensive review series)
  Bibliography: p.
  Includes index.
  1. Medical technology. I. Title. [DNLM:
1. Technology, Medical—Examination questions.
QY18 C737]
RB37.S38 1979   616′.002′02   78-31823
ISBN 0-8016-4487-9

C/M/M 9 8 7 6 5 4 3 2 1   02/C/279

Contributors

EDWIN LEWIS BEMIS, M.D., F.C.A.P., F.A.S.C.P.

Associate Director of Laboratories and Vice Chief of Medical
Staff, Deaconess Hospital; Assistant Clinical Professor of
Pathology, Medical College of Wisconsin; Lecturer in Medical
Technology, Marquette University, Milwaukee, Wisconsin

ANTHONY CAFARO, M.D., F.C.A.P., F.A.S.C.P.

Associate Pathologist, St. Joseph's Hospital; Lecturer in Medical
Technology, Marquette University, Milwaukee, Wisconsin

SILAS G. FARMER, Ph.D.

Microbiologist, Milwaukee County Medical Complex; Associate
Professor of Pathology, Medical College of Wisconsin; Clinical
Professor of Mibrobiology, Marquette University School of
Dentistry; Fellow, American Academy of Microbiology; Diplomate,
American Board of Medical Microbiology; Lecturer in Medical
Technology, Marquette University, Milwaukee, Wisconsin

OPAL KELLY, M.T.(ASCP)

Medical Technologist Supervisor, Milwaukee County Medical
Complex; Lecturer in Medical Technology, Marquette University,
Milwaukee, Wisconsin

RICHARD A. KOMOROWSKI, M.D., F.A.S.C.P.

Associate Professor of Pathology, Medical College of Wisconsin;
Pathologist, Milwaukee County Medical Complex; Lecturer in Medical
Technology, Marquette University, Milwaukee, Wisconsin

GORDON E. LANG, M.D., F.C.A.P., F.A.S.C.P.

Associate Pathologist, St. Mary's Hospital; Lecturer in Medical
Technology, Marquette University, Milwaukee, Wisconsin

ALFRED MEYERS, M.D., F.C.A.P., F.A.S.C.P.

Associate Pathologist, St. Mary's Hospital; Assistant Clinical
Professor in Pathology, Medical College of Wisconsin; Lecturer in
Medical Technology, Marquette University, Milwaukee, Wisconsin

JOHN D. REEVES, M.S., M.T.(ASCP)

Instrumentation Quality Assurance Coordinator, Department of Pathology,
Mount Sinai Medical Center, Milwaukee, Wisconsin

JOAN SHROUT, M.S., M.T.(ASCP) C.

Assistant Education Coordinator, School of Medical
Technology, Mount Sinai Medical Center, Milwaukee, Wisconsin

RAYMOND ZASTROW, M.Ed., M.D., F.C.A.P.

Pathologist and Director of Radio-chemistry, St. Michael's
Hospital; Assistant Clinical Professor of Pathology, Medical
College of Wisconsin; Lecturer in Medical Technology, Marquette
University, Milwaukee, Wisconsin; Member, American College of
Nuclear Physicians; Member, American College of Nuclear Medicine

Preface

Upon arriving at the close of academic preparation for a career as a medical laboratory technologist, a student will have reached a career milestone. College and clinical education (internship) is designed to prepare each student to be a competent technologist. The next goal is certification or licensure. This book was written to help the reader review the academic background so that this goal can be achieved successfully.

This book is intended only as a review mechanism. It does not provide detailed explanations. Students should consider the questions contained herein, determine whether they understand the concepts and facts presented, and return to their textbooks and personal notes for further study as needed.

We have not dealt with methodology but with the understanding of laboratory procedures and their pathophysiologic ramifications. The student should not memorize such details of procedures as amounts of reagents used but should concentrate on their sequence in the procedure and the reason for their use. To help the student review, we have included outlines that may be used as study guides. Also included is a listing of procedures that the student should have studied throughout the year of clinical work. This listing represents the type of procedures one would find available to the physicians on the staff of a modern, average-sized, urban hospital, short of the status of a research center. By referring to the list of procedures and asking the questions contained in the appropriate outlines, the student should have an organized method of review.

The education of medical laboratory technologists extends beyond that of medical laboratory technicians so that they may not only perform laboratory procedures but may also be able to correlate, interpret, compare, and analyze them. The questions in this book were devised to assist in achieving this objective.

The student should not be apprehensive regarding the mechanics and the format of the examinations. Frequently there is more than one possible answer. Since the best choice is the most correct answer, the examinee should be careful to analyze all choices before selecting the final answer.

Examinees who feel great anxiety over the examination should purchase a handbook on how to take an examination. These are available in most college or university bookstores. The AMA-approved hospital that graduated the student did so with the conviction that he or she would successfully pass the certification or licensure examination. Achieving a passing score on an examination that leads to successful certification or licensure is only part of the medical technologist's goal. Technical competence must accompany successful certification or licensure for those who wish to practice as professional medical laboratory technologists. It is appropriate to begin this review with an honest self-assessment of one's technical competence. The review should be started 6 weeks before an examination is to be taken. Those having doubts regarding their technical competence should return to their practicum teachers in the laboratory to review techniques. Without technical competence, academic competence is of little value in the laboratory.

Because of the rising trend to make continuing education a contingency for continued certification and licensure, we hope that this book will serve as a source of reference for persons seeking insight into current theories and practices in the medical laboratory. In addition to senior medical technology students, the following individuals will find this book helpful: (1) practicing technologists who wish to update their information either in the area of medical technology in which they are currently engaged or in an area to which they wish to transfer their interest, (2) technologists wishing to return to work after a number of years of absence from the laboratory, or (3) persons wishing to prepare for academic equivalency examinations given by the College-Level Examination Program (CLEP) of the College Entrance Examination Board, Princeton, New Jersey.

This book is the result of the cooperative effort of many. We have attempted to give the student or examinee a concise guide for study. This second edition of the book represents an updating of much of the material. We have made no attempt to present a simulated examination because the medical technologist may select from a number of examinations to attain certification or licensure. Each examination has a different testing approach, but all are based on the assumption that the student has an understanding of the principles (physical, chemical, or biologic) involved in the practice of medical laboratory technology. Thus, we hope that the student is stimulated to pursue the subject matter included herein in a manner not of memorization but of understanding.

Alice M. Semrad

Study guide for students

CLINICAL MICROBIOLOGY

A. Name and classification of infectious agent
B. Methodology
   1. Collection and handling of specimen
     a. Source of specimen
     b. Aseptic technique required
   2. Identification
     a. Cellular morphology and staining
     b. Colonial characteristics
     c. Growth requirements
       (1) Nutritional (known media components and the reason for their use)
         (a) For isolation
         (b) For differentiation
       (2) Atmospheric
   3. Serologic reactions
   4. Antibiotic susceptibility
C. Pathogenicity
   1. Pathologic process resulting from infection
     a. Relationship of process to laboratory findings (serology, hematology, chemistry)
     b. Immunologic response
   2. Transmission
   3. Epidemiology

CLINICAL CHEMISTRY

A. Name of substance to be analyzed
   1. Chemical classification of compound
   2. Reference method
   3. Routine chemical method
B. Methodology

1. Outline the procedure step by step, including:
   a. How to obtain the specimen
   b. How to preserve the specimen
2. Discuss the chemistry of the procedure, i.e., the purpose of each step and chemistry involved (when a particular instrument is used, discuss it and its application)
3. Sources of errors in the procedure (endogenous and exogenous)
4. Quality control
5. Quality assurance
6. Contraindications in using the procedure
7. Advantages and disadvantages of the procedure
C. Pathophysiology
1. The normal physiologic and biochemical relationships of the substance with related anatomy
2. Conditions in the patient resulting in variations in the physiology and biochemistry leading to abnormal values (high or low)
3. Relationship of this substance to other laboratory findings

CLINICAL MICROSCOPY*

A. Choice of type of microscopy and light source
B. Preparation of the material to be viewed
C. Characteristics to be examined:
1. Size
2. Shape
3. Symmetry
4. Thickness (e.g., third dimension or depth of form)
5. Consistency (e.g., light transmission)
6. Constituents or components (e.g., structural units)
7. Movement (if any)

PROCEDURES FOR CHEMISTRY

Acid phosphatase	Blood gases and electrolytes
Albumin	pH
Albumin-binding capacity	P_{CO_2}
Alcohol level	P_{O_2}
Alkaline phosphatase	P_{50}
Ammonia	CO
Amylase	CO_2
Barbiturate level	% Oxygen saturation
Bilirubin	Osmolality measurement

---

*This outline can be used whether it be the microscopic study of urinary sediment, blood smears for hematologic studies, or microbiologic studies.

Chloride
Lithium
Potassium
Sodium
BSP
BUN
Calcium
Cholesterol
CPK
Creatinine
Creatinine clearance
Diagnex blue
2,3-DPG
Gamma glutamyl transferase
  (GGT)
Gastric analysis
Glucose
Hemoglobin

Iron-binding capacity
Iron serum
Lactate levels
LDH
Lipase
Lipids (total)
Magnesium
5′ Nucleotidase
Phosphorus (inorganic)
Protein (total)
PSP
Salicylate level
Serotonin
SGOT
SGPT
Stone analysis
Triglyceride
Uric acid

PROCEDURES FOR COAGULATION

Circulating anticoagulant tests
Clot retraction
Correction of abnormal prothrombin
  time
Duke bleeding time
Euglobulin clot lysis
Factor assay (intrinsic and extrinsic)
Fibrin split products
Fibrin stabilizing factor, 5M urea
  test for
Fibrinogen assay
Heparin neutralization
Ivy bleeding time
Lee-White whole blood clotting time

Make-up corrective plasmas and
  serum
Partial thromboplastin time
Plasma recalcification time
Platelet screening
Protamine paracoagulation
Prothrombin consumption time
Prothrombin time
Reptilase time
Rumple-Leede test
Stypven time
Thrombin time
Thromboplastin generation time

PROCEDURES FOR HEMATOLOGY

Autohemolysin test
Bone marrow prep
Cytogenetics
  Culture
  Karyotyping
Differential counts—peripheral and
  bone marrow

Electrophoresis—hemoglobin,
  haptoglobin
Fragility tests—osmotic, mechanical,
  acid
Giemsa stain
G-6-PDH—assay, fluorescent,
  ascorbate-cyanide

Heinz body stain
Hematocrit
Hemoglobin
Histiocyte smear
Indices calculation
Kliehauer stain
LE—standard, fluorescent
Leukocyte alkaline phosphatase stain
Malaria smears (thick and thin)
Mechanical fragility
Nasal smear for eosinophils
Nitroblue tetrazolium stain
Osmotic fragility

Particle counts
Automated
Manual (WBC, RBC, platelets,
eosinophils, and sperm)
Periodic acid–Schiff stain
Peroxidase stain
Reticulocyte count
Sedimentation rate
Sickle cell preparation
Sickledex
Spinal fluid cell count
Sudan black B stain
Wright's stain

PROCEDURES FOR IMMUNOHEMATOLOGY

ABO typing
ABO typing discrepancies
Absorption elution
Amniocentesis
Antenatal workup
Antibody screening
Antigen typing and identification
Component therapy
Coombs testing
Cord blood studies
Crossmatch
Du testing

Family studies
Genotyping
Hemolysis A and B
Identification panel
Immune A and B titer
Incompatible crossmatch
Leukagglutinins
Rh titration
Rh typing
RhoGam procedure
Subgrouping
Transfusion reaction

PROCEDURES FOR SEROLOGY

Alpha antitrypsin
Alpha fetoglobin
Amebiasis
Antihyaluronidase
ASO titer
C reactive protein
Cold agglutinins
Complement levels
Erythropoietin levels
Febrile agglutination
Fibrin split products
Hemagglutination inhibition
Histoplasmosis

Leptospirosis
Migratory inhibition factor
Monospot
Neuramidase
Rheumatoid arthritis
RPR
Rubella
T cells
Thyroid antibody test
Toxoplasmosis
Trichinosis
VDRL

INFECTIOUS AGENTS FOR BACTERIOLOGY*

Micrococcus
Staphylococcus
Gaffkya, Aerococcus
Streptococcus
*Enterococcus (Streptococcus
faecalis)*
*Pneumococcus (Streptococcus
pneumoniae)*
Neisseria
Pseudomonas
Moraxella
Acinetobacter
Flavobacterium
Xanthomonas
Alcaligenes
Escherichia
Shigella
Edwardsiella
Salmonella
Arizona
Citrobacter
Klebsiella
Enterobacter
Serratia
Proteus
Yersinia
Vibrio, Campylobacter
Haemophilus

Bordetella
Brucella
Pasteurella
Francisella
Bacillus
Corynebacterium
Listeria
Erysipelothrix
Clostridium
Bifidobacterium
Propionibacterium
Eubacterium
Lactobacillus
Actinomyces
Arachnia
Bacteroides
Fusobacterium
Peptococcus
Peptostreptococcus
Veillonella
Mycobacterium
Spirillum
Borrelia
Treponema
Leptospira
Aeromonas
Streptobacillus
Mycoplasma

INFECTIOUS AGENTS FOR PARASITOLOGY†

Cestodes
  Diphyllobothrium latum
  Dipylidium caninum
  Echinococcus granulosus
  Echinococcus multilocularis
  Hymenolepis diminuta
  Hymenolepis nana
  Taenia saginata
  Taenia solium

Nematodes
  Acanthocheilonema perstans
  Ancylostoma braziliense
  Ancylostoma duodenale
  Ascaris lumbricoides
  Enterobius vermicularis
  Loa loa
  Mansonella ozzardi
  Necator americanus

---

*Identify the clinically significant species of the following genera.
†Identify the clinically significant stages.

Onchocerca volvulus
Strongyloides stercoralis
Toxocara canis
Toxocara cati
Trichinella spiralis
Trichuris trichiura
Wuchereria bancrofti
Wuchereria malayi
Protozoa
Balantidium coli
Chilomastix mesnili
Dientamoeba fragilis
Endolimax nana
Entamoeba coli
Entamoeba gingivalis
Entamoeba histolytica
Giardia lamblia
Iodamoeba buetschlii
Leishmania braziliensis
Leishmania donovani
Leishmania tropica

Plasmodium falciparum
Plasmodium malariae
Plasmodium ovale
Plasmodium vivax
Toxoplasma gondii
Trichomonas hominis
Trichomonas tenax
Trichomonas vaginalis
Trypanosoma cruzi
Trypanosoma gambiense
Trypanosoma rhodesiense
Trematodes
Clonorchis sinensis
Fasciola hepatica
Fasciolopsis buski
Heterophyes heterophyes
Paragonimus westermani
Schistosoma dermatitis
Schistosoma haematobium
Schistosoma japonicum
Schistosoma mansoni

PROCEDURES FOR URINALYSIS

Physical properties
  Physical appearance
  Specific gravity
Chemical properties
  Bilirubin
  Glucose
  Ketones
  Occult blood
  pH
  Protein
  Crystal identification

Aminoacidurias
Bence Jones protein
Calcium
Hemosiderin
Homogentisic acid
Human chorionic gonadotropin
Melanin
Porphobilinogen
Addis count
Concentration and dilution tests

PROCEDURES FOR STOOL ANALYSIS

Fat
Meat fibers
Occult blood

Starch
Trypsin

Contents

CHAPTER 1

Hemostasis

Edwin Lewis Bemis

■ **Give a simple classification of the hemorrhagic disorders.**

There are two general types: *primary* disorders, which are usually congenital (present at birth), often familial or hereditary, and presumably due to a genetic defect; and *secondary* disorders, which are acquired and related to some other underlying disease. Whether primary or secondary, they may be most simply classified as dependent on a defect of the supportive tissues about blood vessels, of the blood vessels themselves, of blood platelets, or of blood plasma. However, recent knowledge indicates that there are many combined defects, as will be illustrated in some of the following.

■ **Give examples of extravascular (tissue) bleeding disorders.**

The Ehlers-Danlos syndrome is a hereditary disorder associated with marked hyperelasticity and fragility of the skin along with defective aggregation of platelets to collagen. Acquired abnormalities include senile purpura, which is associated with degenerative changes of supportive tissues, and postmenopausal purpura, which is as yet poorly understood.

■ **Give examples of vascular bleeding disorders.**

Hereditary telangiectasia, or Rendu-Osler disease, is a genetic disorder that is transmitted as a dominant trait and is characterized by the presence of dilated capillaries and venules on mucous membranes, often in clusters, that are usually first noted in adult life. The vascular dilatations may be due to abnormal connective tissue within or outside the vessel walls. The surface location of such clusters predisposes to bleeding, frequently secondary to extraneous or environmental factors such as alcohol, various drugs of which aspirin is an example, and, in a few subjects, exposure to sunlight. The tourniquet test is abnormal in a high percentage of such cases. Of course, the most obvious

1

example of *acquired* vascular bleeding is injury that causes loss of integrity of blood vessels, allowing blood to leak out (as in trauma, often surgically induced). Other acquired disorders include syphilis and arteriosclerosis, in which rupture of an aneurysm is the common hemorrhagic manifestation. Acquired vascular purpura may also be associated with a wide variety of agents that increase the permeability of the vessel lining (endothelium), resulting in petechiae and purpura. Such disorders include damage from immunologic reactions, termed "allergic vasculitis," of which Schönlein-Henoch purpura is one type; conditions associated with obstruction of vessels such as sometimes occurs when there are abnormal proteins (e.g., cryoglobulins) or bacteria (e.g., meningococci) in the blood; and vitamin C deficiency (scurvy), because this vitamin is required to maintain the cement substance (hyaluronic acid) between endothelial cells.

■ **What is the relationship between vascular purpura, pseudohemophilia, the Minot–von Willebrand syndrome, and von Willebrand's disease?**

These are all terms that have been used to designate the same condition, which is perhaps the *most common hereditary hemorrhagic disease known* and therefore of extreme importance. It was first described in 1920 by Minot and in 1926 by von Willebrand and is characteristically transmitted as an autosomal dominant trait, appearing in both males and females in about equal proportions but with variable penetrance. It was first attributed to some unknown vascular abnormality and was defined in the laboratory only by a prolonged bleeding time. Present knowledge indicates that severely afflicted individuals have little or no factor VIII–related antigen in either their endothelial cells or their platelets and that there is an abnormality of a plasma protein related to factor VIII (antihemophilic globulin) that is necessary for platelets to form normal adhesion to connective tissue. It is still not known precisely how this von Willebrand factor (VWF) activity of factor VIII interacts with platelets.

■ **What laboratory test abnormalities may be seen in patients with von Willebrand's disease?**

There is a wide spectrum, with variability in both clinical expression and laboratory findings. Test abnormalities include a prolonged bleeding time; reduced factor VIII activity by assay; reduced, low-normal, or aberrant factor VIII–related antigen; abnormal platelet retention in a glass bead column; defective ristocetin-induced platelet aggregation (or agglutination) that corrects with purified factor VIII or with normal plasma; and overresponse of factor VIII activity levels after transfusion with normal plasma, hemophilic plasma, or factor VIII concentrates.

■ **How may bleeding disorders due to platelet abnormalities be classified?**

In addition to being divided into primary and secondary disorders, they should be further classified into those that are associated with a quantitative, decreased number of platelets *(thrombocytopenia)* and those that are associated with a qualitative, *functional* abnormality (irrespective of number).

■ **Are the primary abnormalities of platelets common?**

No, they are extremely rare. The primary disorders are all *congenital,* and most have been associated with decreased numbers of megakaryocytes. Congenital thrombocytopenia may be due to *defective or decreased production* (as in Fanconi's syndrome, congenital leukemia, maternal rubella, maternal ingestion of thiazide diuretics, and deficiency of thrombopoietin). Increased platelet *destruction* may be of a *nonimmune* nature, as occurs in association with hemolytic disease of the newborn or with infection, or of an *immune* nature, as occurs in association with maternal drug sensitivity, maternal idiopathic thrombocytopenia, or isoimmune neonatal thrombocytopenia (which, although uncommon, is a life-threatening situation that requires immediate transfusion with washed maternal platelets or exchange transfusion). Congenital *qualitative* platelet abnormalities are perhaps the least common of all, but many have been characterized by recently developed tests for platelet function. Functional abnormalities are often referred to as thrombocytopathic states or thrombopathies, whether congenital or acquired. The congenital thrombopathies associated with *defective platelet aggregation* include Glanzmann's thrombasthenia (defective sensitivity to ADP and markedly defective clot retraction), storage pool disease (decreased content of ADP, ATP, serotonin, and calcium), the Wiskott-Aldrich syndrome (decreased content of ADP and defective phagocytosis), afibrinogenemia, and many more that are often associated with other congenital abnormalities. The Bernard-Soulier syndrome is characterized by a combination of thrombocytopenia and defective ristocetin-induced aggregation along with the presence of giant platelets.

■ **What are the most common causes of hemorrhagic disease?**

The secondary, acquired disorders of platelets are the most com-

mon causes and are therefore also extremely important. Decreased numbers of platelets may be due to diminished production or increased removal from the circulation. Examination of bone marrow for the presence of megakaryocytes usually permits a distinction. *Thrombocytopenia* may result from sequestration in an enlarged spleen (hypersplenism), from excessive loss during extracorporeal bypass surgical procedures, from hypothermia, or following multiple transfusions of stored (platelet-poor) blood. *Defective or decreased production* may be secondary to infiltrative disease of the marrow, radiation or drug exposure, paroxysmal nocturnal hemoglobinuria (PNH), idiopathic aplastic anemia, nutritional deficiency, or cyclic thrombocytopenia. *Increased destruction or removal* may be on a *nonimmune* basis and secondary to infection (gram-negative sepsis), disseminated intravascular coagulation (DIC), the hemolytic-uremic syndrome, drugs (ristocetin, heparin?) or thrombotic thrombocytopenic purpura (TTP, angiopathic thrombohemolytic thrombocytopenia, or Moschcowitz's disease). Increased destruction of an *immune* nature may be drug-induced (e.g., quinine, quinidine), may follow transfusions (posttransfusion purpura), or may occur for unknown reasons (idiopathic thrombocytopenia purpura [ITP], acute postinfectious and chronic forms). *Acquired functional* platelet abnormalities (thrombopathies) are most commonly due to defective ADP release (with aggregation defects) in association with drug ingestion (e.g., aspirin, dipyridamole [Persantin], antihistaminics, and tranquilizers), renal failure, liver disease, or fibrinolytic states. In polycythemia vera, essential thrombocythemia, some instances of chronic granulocytic leukemia, and myelofibrosis, there may be a functional abnormality despite markedly elevated numbers of platelets.

■ **How are platelets involved in primary and secondary hemostasis?**

Platelets are essential for the formation of white thrombi, or primary hemostatic plugs, which seal gaps in damaged blood vessels through a sequence of reactions that constitute the body's first line of defense against blood loss. *Primary hemostasis* involves two stages, which are reversible unless followed by consolidation of the plug, action of thrombin, and definitive formation of fibrin (which is *secondary hemostasis*). These first two stages involve platelet adhesion and aggregation. Following trauma to a vessel, platelets adhere to exposed collagen fibers of connective tissue (recall that VWF is a necessary cofactor for this reaction). Platelets then swell, extend pseudopodia, lose some of their granular constituents, and selectively release ADP, serotonin, catecholamines (notably epinephrine), and platelet factor 4 (a highly basic protein with antiheparin activity). ADP released from the dense granules of platelets and from the damaged tissue affects other platelets in the vicinity and causes them to release additional ADP (initiating the amplification step or secondary wave of platelet aggregation). With further aggregation and consolidation of platelets, platelet phospholipid factor 3 is released and interacts with plasma coagulation factors to convert fibrinogen to fibrin (the *intrinsic pathway* of coagulation). This results in still further aggregation and shrinking of platelets into solidly fused masses, with the development of fibrin at the periphery of the plug and in channels traversing it.

■ **How is coagulation initiated in vitro?**

It may be initiated by contact with glass and, following the intrinsic pathway, results first in the formation of plasma thromboplastin. If initiated by *preformed* tissue thromboplastin in the presence of calcium, this first "stage" is avoided and coagulation proceeds following the *extrinsic pathway* (dependent on factor VII, which is not required in the intrinsic pathway). In either pathway there next follows the conversion of prothrombin to thrombin and then the conversion of fibrinogen to fibrin monomers, which are polymerized in the presence of factor XIII to form an insoluble clot.

■ **Is the cascade, or waterfall, theory of coagulation valid?**

This hypothesis states that each plasma factor is converted to its active form by the preceding factor in a kind of chain reaction, as illustrated in the diagram at the end of this chapter. More recent studies have indicated that factors V and VIII form complexes involving activated proteins, calcium ions, and phospholipids contributed by the platelets. These complexes in turn convert the next factor in the cascade to an active enzyme.

■ **Which plasma factor deficiencies may be associated with abnormal hemostasis and clinical bleeding?**

A deficiency of any factor (with the exceptions of factor XII, the Fletcher factor, or the Fitzgerald factor) may be associated with abnormal hemostasis and clinical bleeding. Although congenital deficiencies of these proteins may cause abnormal clotting in vitro, such deficiencies are not usually associated with clinical bleeding.

■ **What is the importance of kinins?**

The complexity of the coagulation system has grown with the recent discovery of abnormalities in prekallikrein (the Fletcher factor) and high–molecular weight kininogen (the Fitzgerald factor). Kinins are important in the inflammatory response, but in addition, recent evidence indicates that prekallikrein may be the plasminogen proactivator. Kallikrein has also been implicated in the activation of factor XII.

■ **What is the importance of physiologic anticoagulants?**

The importance of alpha-1-antitrypsin, alpha-2-macroglobulin, and antithrombin III has only recently been appreciated. Except for factors V, VIII, and XIII, the coagulation proteins circulate as inactive factors, which are converted to serine proteases. These proteases may be inhibited by the plasma anticoagulants, of which the most important is *antithrombin III (the heparin cofactor)*. Antithrombin III inhibits not only many of the clotting factors but also plasmin and kallikrein. Inhibition is accelerated by the presence of heparin, which seems to bind to antithrombin III, altering its molecular configuration so as to cause inactivation at the serine site of the coagulant proteins. Hereditary deficiency of antithrombin III results in a high incidence of deep vein thrombosis. In major thromboembolic diseases, antithrombin III levels are often reduced. Women receiving oral contraceptives, particularly those with a high estrogen content, also have decreased antithrombin III levels. Heparin is not an effective anticoagulant in the absence of antithrombin III, and some cases of clinical heparin failure may be due to a deficiency of this substance (as in chronic DIC).

■ **Classify bleeding disorders due to hereditary plasma factor deficiencies.**

This may be easily done according to the "stage" of coagulation altered by their absence. Any hereditary deficiency of a thromboplastinogenic factor is referred to as *true hemophilia*, which afflicts one person in 10,000 of the world population. Classical *hemophilia A* (deficiency of AHG, AHF, factor VIII) is five times more common than *hemophilia B* (Christmas disease, deficiency of PTC, factor IX). Both are transmitted by female carriers and affect males predominantly (sex-linked, recessive Mendelian trait), but in about 30% of cases there is no traceable family history. The disease is extremely serious and is noted for the spontaneous occurrence of hemorrhages into joints (hemarthroses). Patients with this disease usually have a normal bleeding time (unlike those with von Willebrand's disease). Rare cases of hemophilia are due to a lack of PTA (factor XI). Hereditary plasma factor deficiencies associated with thrombogenesis are rare,

are all apparently transmitted as simple Mendelian recessive traits, and are associated with bleeding resembling that of mild hemophilia. Hereditary deficiency of labile factor V is termed parahemophilia, or Owren's disease. Hereditary afibrinogenemia and lack of fibrin stabilizing factor (XIII) are even more uncommon.

■ **How do bleeding disorders due to acquired plasma factor deficiencies differ from the hereditary plasma factor disorders?**

Secondary or acquired disorders are usually due to *multiple* deficiencies of plasma factors rather than to the single defects typical of the hereditary disorders. Such multiple defects often form characteristic patterns that reflect the underlying abnormality responsible for them. Examples include primary liver disease, vitamin K deficiency states, DIC with secondary excess circulating fibrinolysins, primary excess fibrinolysis, and circulating anticoagulants.

■ **What factor assay may be helpful in distinguishing bleeding due to hepatic disease from that due to vitamin K deficiency?**

An assay of factor V, which is produced in the liver independent of the presence of vitamin K. Clinical response to the parenteral administration of vitamin K (with shortening of prothrombin times in vitamin K deficiency states) is probably used more often, particularly when the patient has been taking a coumarin drug as an anticoagulant, since such drugs are antagonistic to the vitamin.

■ **What are some other causes of vitamin K deficiency?**

Defective synthesis by intestinal bacteria, poor absorption from the bowel, and lack of utilization by the liver. Prolonged treatment with antibiotics may diminish bacterial synthesis. Conditions obstructing the flow of bile may cause decreased absorption and may be associated with vitamin K deficiency as well as obstructive jaundice. Hemorrhagic disease of the newborn, caused by vitamin K deficiency, is probably due to a combination of decreased synthesis and deficient absorption (bleeding in the newborn is not always due to vitamin K deficiency).

■ **What is the relationship between the defibrination syndrome, DIC, and consumption coagulopathy?**

These are all terms used to denote the same hemorrhagic disorder, which is caused by widespread clotting in small blood vessels throughout the body. Certain plasma coagulation factors (I, II, V, and VIII) are "consumed" along with platelets, and plasminogen is also activated (secondary fibrinolysis), with the release of fibrin monomers as well as fibrinogen degradation products (fragments X, Y, D, and E) into the circulation (the degradation products also exert an anticoagulant effect). The clotting is probably generated by the release of thromboplastic substances and is seen in association with such conditions as premature separation of the placenta, septic abortion, surgical trauma, hemolytic transfusion reactions, and the myeloproliferative disorders.

■ **Why is DIC often difficult to distinguish from primary excess fibrinolysis?**

Both are associated with clot lysis, the release of fibrinogen degradation and fibrin split products, and abnormalities of multiple tests for coagulation (the demonstration of *decreased platelets and fibrin monomers* in DIC helps to distinguish between the two). It is important to remember that DIC is always a secondary disorder and that treatment of the underlying disease must be given prime consideration.

■ **Does DIC occur without associated bleeding?**

Yes, perhaps even more commonly than with an overt acute hemorrhagic diathesis and in both subacute and chronic forms (e.g., in most patients with disseminated malignancy). Here, slow activation of clotting is attended by an increased production (as well as utilization) of clotting factors. Although fibrinogen degradation and fibrin split products may be demonstrable, there may also be very high fibrinogen levels and platelet counts as well as "better than normal" tests for coagulation (PCT, PTT, PT).

■ **How is bleeding caused by endogenous circulating anticoagulants?**

Some may specifically inhibit one coagulation factor (e.g., anti–factor VIII following repeated administration of cryoprecipitate), whereas others have more general anticoagulant properties. Some are abnormal proteins that develop during the course of malignant disease, such as macroglobulins and cryoglobulins (dysproteinemias), and apparently interfere with proper polymerization of fibrin. A specific anti–factor X has been occasionally reported in association with disseminated lupus erythematosus. Still others are "heparinlike" and may be counteracted by the administration of protamine.

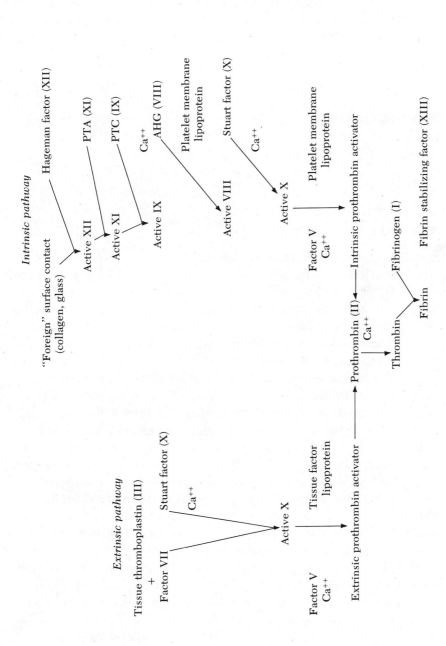

CHAPTER 2

Hematology

The erythrocytes

EDWIN LEWIS BEMIS

■ What is extramedullary hemopoiesis?

Extramedullary hemopoiesis refers to production of blood cells by organs other than the bone marrow, notably the spleen. It may occur whenever the bone marrow is replaced by abnormal tissue (e.g., in myelosclerosis with myeloid metaplasia) or whenever the bone marrow fails to supply an increased demand for cells.

■ What is the function of erythrocytes?

Erythrocytes provide suitable vehicles for the synthesis, transport, and protection of hemoglobin molecules, which are capable of accepting, transporting, and delivering oxygen to all tissues of the body.

■ What are the basic elements required for hemoglobin synthesis?

Protoporphyrin III, an adequate amount of iron in a usable form, "hemopoietic factors" (vitamin B_{12}, folate, vitamin C, hormones) for normal orderly cell maturation, and globin with the necessary polypeptide chains are the elements required for hemoglobin synthesis.

■ What are some disease states that may be associated with variations in the erythrocyte sedimentation rate?

In polycythemia with a high volume of packed red cells the sedimentation rate is extremely slow, as it is in the blood of the newborn; slow rates are characteristically found in sickle cell anemia as well. Increased rates of sedimentation are found in the presence of increased quantities of proteins of high molecular weight, such as fibrinogen in association with various inflammatory processes, or in dysproteinemia (e.g., with plasma cell myeloma).

■ **What are the changes that occur as red and white blood cells mature?**

They are reduction in the size of the cell as well as its nucleus, loss of nucleoli, and signs of differentiation (hemoglobin formation and extrusion of nucleus in erythrocytes or segmentation of nuclei with formation of specific granules in the cytoplasm of granulocytes).

■ **What are some of the tests that may be altered "fictitiously" by recent blood transfusions?**

Donor red cells may alter any test that is dependent on examination of the patient's red cells alone, for example, hemoglobin electrophoresis, the 1-minute alkali denaturation test for fetal hemoglobin, and tests for glucose-6-phosphate dehydrogenase (G-6-PD) deficiency and pyruvic kinase deficiency.

■ **How long after a blood transfusion may the bone marrow in pernicious anemia convert from a megaloblastic to a normoblastic character?**

This usually occurs within several hours; this is also the case following an injection of vitamin B_{12}.

■ **What are the cellular structural elements concerned with hemoglobin synthesis?**

The mitochondria are involved in porphyrin synthesis, and heme is formed with the incorporation of iron from ferritin aggregates in the cell; globin synthesis takes place in the ribosomes of the endoplasmic reticulum.

■ **What laboratory features may lead poisoning have in common with porphyria?**

The excretion of delta aminolevulinic acid, porphobilinogen, and other abnormal porphyrins, along with protoporphyrin fluorescence of erythrocytes, are some manifestations of lead poisoning.

■ **What are some of the likely diagnoses in a patient having normocytic, normochromic anemia and an elevated platelet count?**

Acute blood loss and an underlying malignancy are probably the most commonly encountered conditions.

■ **What do you know about the iron-binding capacity of blood?**

Normally, iron-binding protein (transferrin) is present in quantities sufficient to bind about $300\mu g$ of iron per 100 ml plasma; usually this is only one-third saturated with iron. Serum iron concentration shows a distinct diurnal variation (highest in the morning and lowest in the late evening) in the normal person, but this variation is minimal in the presence of a hematologic disorder. Iron-binding capacity is remarkably constant in the normal person.

■ **What is the difference between hemosiderosis and hemochromatosis?**

The presence of large amounts of storage iron in body tissues, unattended by tissue damage, is called hemosiderosis. Hemochromatosis is a disorder in which excessive amounts of iron in the body are associated with damage to the tissues, frequently resulting in cirrhosis of the liver and diabetes mellitus.

■ **What amount of hemoglobin may be synthesized from normal body iron stores?**

When iron metabolism is normal, adult body stores are usually sufficient for the synthesis of about 210 gm of hemoglobin or about 1,500 ml of blood.

■ **What is anemia?**

Anemia is a condition in which there is a reduced concentration of hemoglobin in the peripheral blood, with an associated decrease of oxygen-carrying capacity and symptoms resulting therefrom. Anemia is not always attended by a reduction in the number of circulating erythrocytes.

■ **What may cause an anemia associated with microcytic, hypochromic red cells and a normoblastic bone marrow?**

The cause may be an iron deficiency state, most commonly associated with chronic blood loss in patients from the United States. Newborns have an increased need for iron, particularly during the first 6 months of life, and, unless given supplements, are also prone to develop this form of anemia.

■ **What is pyridoxine-responsive anemia?**

Pyridoxine-responsive anemia is a microcytic, hypochromic anemia that is associated with adequate iron storage and elevated serum iron level and that responds to pyridoxine (vitamin B_6) therapy.

■ **What is hemopoietic principle?**

It is that substance required for the normal, orderly maturation of blood cells, including those of the myeloid and megakaryocytic series as well as red cells. The major factors embodied in hemopoietic principle include vitamin B_{12} and folic acid (folate). A deficiency of either factor may produce megaloblastic dyspoiesis and pancytopenia.

■ **What is pernicious anemia?**

Pernicious anemia is a chronic illness resulting from lack of intrinsic factor in gastric secretions, which is necessary for absorption of vitamin B_{12} in the ileum; it may be associated with subacute combined degeneration of the spinal cord as well as megaloblastic dyspoiesis of the bone marrow and pancytopenia. It may be genetically determined in some cases.

■ **What is the Schilling test?**

It is a test for pernicious anemia. Individuals with this disease will not absorb an appreciable amount of an oral dose of radioactive vitamin B_{12} without the prior addition of intrinsic factor.

■ **What is the relationship between diet and reduced serum levels of folate?**

Folic acid polyglutamates (folates) are widely distributed in a variety of foods and are converted to monoglutamates before absorption in the upper one third of the small intestine. Reduced serum levels of folate may occur after only 3 weeks of a folate-deficient diet.

■ **Why is it important to note the presence of hypersegmented neutrophils?**

This may be the first sign of the development of a megaloblastic process in the marrow, particularly in macrocytic anemia of pregnancy.

■ **Can parasitic infestation result in megaloblastic dyspoiesis?**

Yes, notably the presence of *Dibothriocephalus latus* (fish tapeworm) infestation.

■ **When can macrocytosis be seen unassociated with a true macrocytic anemia?**

Macrocytosis is seen as a "normal" finding in the blood of newborns; it is artificially produced by making a blood smear on a nonwettable surface (e.g., siliconized); and it appears when many reticulocytes are present, since reticulocytes are larger than older RBCs.

■ **What are the normal dimers of globins?**

$\alpha_2\beta_2$ (hemoglobin A_1), $\alpha_2\gamma_2$ (hemoglobin F), and $\alpha_2\delta_2$ (hemoglobin A_2).

■ **What is a specific characteristic of fetal hemoglobin?**

It is alkali-resistant (because it contains residues of isoleucine). It is also resistant to oxygen reduction.

■ **What elements are necessary to protect hemoglobin from the effects of oxidant drugs?**

G-6-PD and reduced glutathione are particularly necessary. Deficiency of either one will result in hemolysis and methemoglobinemia on exposure to oxidant drugs.

■ **Will a deficiency of pyruvic kinase in RBCs lead to methemoglobinemia?**

No. It may result in a nonspherocytic, hemolytic anemia unattended by methemoglobinemia.

■ **What is the fate of old red cells that break down within the bloodstream?**

Hemoglobin is released and becomes bound at once to a plasma alpha-2 globulin termed "haptoglobin," which prevents renal excretion; this is then taken up by phagocytic reticuloendothelial (RE) cells for processing in the usual manner. Haptoglobin is normally present in quantities sufficient to bind about 50 to 150 mg of free hemoglobin per 100 ml plasma.

■ **What is hemolytic disease?**

Hemolytic disease is any disorder in which the red cell life span is shorter than normal.

■ **What is compensated hemolytic disease?**

The increased rate of destruction is compensated for by augmented erythropoiesis, and there is no anemia.

■ **What is hemolytic anemia?**

When augmented red cell production is unable to compensate for the increased rate of destruction, anemia develops. Normal marrow cannot increase its effective output of hemoglobin more than 6 to 8 times that of usual, so that when erythrocyte survival is reduced to 15 to 20 days ($1/6$ to $1/8$ of normal), anemia develops and many biochemical changes can be predicted.

■ **What is the most commonly used method for determining red cell life span?**

The most common method is one in which red cells are drawn from a patient, "tagged" with radioactive chromium, and either autotransfused or transfused into a compatible recipient and the rate of disappearance is determined by the fall in degree of radioactivity. Normal $T^{1}/_{2}$, or time for half of the radioactivity to disappear, is 25 to 35 days, depending on the anticoagulant used; this is not the expected half-life of 60 days because of elution of chromium and loss of the tracer through the urine at about 1% per day after the first 24 hours. Gastrointestinal blood loss can also be quantitated by this method.

■ **Why is the measurement of bilirubin and urobilinogen not always helpful in assessing a hemolytic process?**

The amount of pigment excreted is proportional not only to the rate of hemoglobin breakdown but also to the amount available. Thus, reduction of erythrocyte survival to one half of normal in a patient with only half the normal amount of circulating hemoglobin will seemingly be associated with a "normal" amount of serum bilirubin. In addition, urobilinogen excretion will be affected by diarrhea, constipation, and other factors.

■ **Why is the jaundice of hemolytic anemia termed "acholuric"?**

The clinical sign of jaundice is usually not apparent until serum bilirubin levels are above 3 or 4 mg/100 ml, when the pigment finds its way into the tissues of eye, skin, and so on. The jaundice of hemolytic anemia is termed "acholuric" because it is associated with increased unconjugated bilirubin, which is not excreted into the urine unless there is obstruction of the flow of bile from the liver after conjugation, as may be produced by liver disease or by the obstruction of a large bile duct (e.g., by a gallstone).

■ **Is the reticulocyte count helpful in appraising the level of red cell production?**

Yes. With a normal RBC life span of 120 days, $1/120$ of the total RBCs are destroyed each day and the same number released into the circulation, reflected by a normal reticulocyte count of 0.5 to 1.5 per 100 RBCs. In hemolytic disease the proportion is increased as a rule. However, occasionally the bone marrow "shuts down," producing an aplastic crisis in which reticulocytes may be veritably nil.

■ **Can you give a simple classification of hemolytic disease?**

This may be based on the location of the defect responsible for the shortening of the RBC life span, whether that be within the cell (intracorpuscular), outside the cell (extracorpuscular), or a combination of both (such as the action of oxidant drugs on red cells deficient in G-6-PD).

■ **How is methemalbumin formed?**

When there is intravascular degradation of hemoglobin in excess of 100 to 135 mg/100 ml (which can be bound by haptoglobin), some is directly degraded to heme and globin. Heme is then oxidized to hematin and bound to albumin to form methemalbumin.

■ **Are spherocytes, ovalocytes, or target cells specific for any form of hemolytic disease?**

No. Spherocytes are characteristic of hereditary spherocytosis but are also seen in most other hemolytic disorders as well, particularly in association with extraerythrocytic abnormalities. In hereditary spherocytosis, and perhaps in no other disorder, the mean corpuscular hemoglobin concentration may be elevated over the "forbidden" figure of

36%. Osmotic fragility is also increased. In hereditary ovalocytosis, elliptocytic cells constitute 90% or more of the red cell population, regardless of whether there is heterozygous or homozygous transmission, but ovalocytes are also commonly seen in the hemoglobinopathies and in hypochromic anemias. Target cells are seen in large numbers in thalassemia but are also characteristic of the hemoglobinopathies; they may also be seen in patients with obstructive jaundice, perhaps because of accumulation of free cholesterol in the red cell membrane. Target cells are associated with decreased osmotic fragility.

■ **What is thalassemia?**

Thalassemia is a hereditary, quantitative disorder of hemoglobin synthesis resulting from deficient production of one of the polypeptide chains of globin and the accumulation of "unused" normal chains. The consequences are precipitation of free chains to form inclusion bodies, red cell membrane damage, shortened red cell survival, and the kinetic picture of ineffective erythropoiesis. In perhaps all forms except alpha chain deficiency, there is also a characteristically *low red cell mean corpuscular volume (MCV)*.

■ **In which types of thalassemia do heterozygotes have elevated levels of fetal hemoglobin?**

In *beta-thalassemia trait*, about half such individuals have 2% to 10% hemoglobin F, and although the rest may have normal amounts of F, the proportion of A_2 hemoglobin is usually twice normal. In *delta beta-thalassemia*, A_2 level may be decreased or normal, whereas the amount of F usually varies between 6% and 25%.

■ **Name other conditions that may be associated with elevated levels of fetal hemoglobin.**

Hereditary persistance of fetal hemoglobin (HPFH) may be associated with levels of 10% to 35%. Elevated levels may also be seen in many other conditions, including pregnancy, anemias of different types, myelophthisic disorders, and even bronchial asthma.

■ **What are the most common hemoglobinopathies?**

That associated with sickle hemoglobin, caused by valine replacement of glutamic acid in residue no. 6 of the beta chains, is perhaps the most common abnormality in the United States, occurring in heterozygous form in about 10% of American blacks. Only about one in 400 persons has an associated anemia. Sickling (tactoid formation on exposure to a reducing agent) is found both in individuals with the trait and in those with a form of sickle cell disease. Hemoglobin C, caused by lysine replacement of glutamic acid in residue no. 6 of the beta chains, is present in about 2% of American blacks in the heterozygous form. The homozygous form, usually associated with mild anemia, is rare. Characteristic hemoglobin C crystals with parallel longitudinal margins and pointed ends may be seen, particularly in the homozygous form and especially if the spleen is removed. Hemoglobin D and hemoglobin G are also fairly common; they have the same migration on electrophoresis as hemoglobin S at a high pH but may be separated at pH 6 utilizing citrate agar. Hemoglobin G is probably more common in the American black than has been heretofore known. Hemoglobin D is seen in people from India and the British Isles particularly. Hemoglobin E has an incidence as high as 12% in people from Southeast Asia. This results from lysine replacement of glutamic acid in residue no. 26 of the beta chains. Hemoglobin E has the same electrophoretic mobility at pH 8.6 on cellulose acetate as hemoglobin A_2, C, and O.

■ **What is the worldwide distribution of thalassemia?**

Although called "Mediterranean anemia," the disease occurs not only in southern Europe but in northern Africa, Asia, and other parts of the world. In the United States it occurs most commonly in blacks, with or without an associated hemoglobinopathy.

■ **What is the relationship of complement to paroxysmal nocturnal hemoglobinuria (PNH)?**

Hemolysis in PNH occurs because of an obscure structural defect that renders a proportion of red cells unusually susceptible to the lytic action of complement. Complement may be activated in such cases by acidified serum (Ham test) or by sucrose. The hemolysis in PNH is not necessarily related to any time of day or night, as was previously thought, nor are all cases of PNH restricted to hemolysis alone (some are associated with thrombocytopenia, leukopenia, or pancytopenia).

■ **What is paroxysmal cold hemoglobinuria (PCH)?**

PCH is a hemolytic disorder associated with an extracorpuscular abnormality in which a Donath-Landsteiner hemolysin is fixed to RBCs at low temperatures, with hemolysis occurring on return to a warm environment.

■ **What is cold hemagglutinin disease?**

This is an autoimmune hemolytic disorder associated with high titers of cold agglutinins. It may occur transiently, as in association with *Mycoplasma* pneumonia, or in a more chronic, idiopathic form. Most cold agglutinins are IgM and have anti-I specificity.

■ **What is autoimmune hemolytic disease of "warm antibody type"?**

Hemolytic disease associated with a positive direct Coombs' test is called the "warm antibody type." This is most often associated with another disease entity such as chronic lymphocytic leukemia, malignant lymphoma, or disseminated lupus erythematosus.

■ **What are Heinz body anemias?**

Heinz body anemias are hemolytic disorders associated with coccoid Heinz bodies in the red cells demonstrable with supravital preparations. These can also be visualized by phase-contrast microscopy but are not stained with the usual Romanowsky dyes. They represent intracellular precipitations of denatured hemoglobin. They may occur in normal persons (less than 1%) and are more obvious when the spleen is absent. Increased susceptibility to Heinz body formation may be seen in association with defects in the activity of one of the normal red cell enzymes, such as in G-6-PD deficiency; in association with defects in the rate of synthesis or in the structure of the hemoglobin molecule, such as in alpha-thalassemia; or in other conditions related to the presence of unstable hemoglobin molecules.

■ **What is cardiac hemolytic disease?**

This is a hemolytic disease associated with a cardiac defect. It is most commonly seen following replacement of heart valves, with hemolysis occurring because of trauma to RBCs in passage through the prosthetic valve. Hemoglobinuria is usually a prominent feature.

■ **What are the anemias of bone marrow failure?**

Those associated with ineffective erythropoiesis, wherein the bone marrow is unable to deliver cells to the peripheral blood. They include aplastic anemia, which is usually associated with leukopenia and thrombocytopenia; hypoplastic anemia, which is a term usually applied when there is a pure red cell defect; sideroblastic anemias, which are associated with large amounts of nonhemoglobin iron in erythrocyte precursors, large iron stores, and high serum iron levels (some such cases are responsive to pyridoxine therapy); anemias caused by metabolic inhibition of the bone marrow, as seen in association with cancer, severe infection, or kidney or liver disease; and so-called myelophthisis, in which there is abnormal tissue in the bone marrow such as cancerous tissue, the fibrous tissue of myelofibrosis, inflammatory tissue associated with tuberculosis, and so on. Myelophthisis is often associated with marked hemopoiesis in extramedullary sites such as the spleen; only about 50% of such cases show anemia. The most characteristic finding is the presence of nucleated RBCs and a few immature leukocytes in the peripheral blood; this has led to the term "leukoerythroblastosis."

■ **What is polycythemia?**

Polycythemia is a term used to indicate an increased concentration of RBCs in the peripheral blood to above the limits of normal (over 5.7 million/mm^3 for females or 6.4 million/mm^3 for males). *Relative polycythemia* refers to an apparent increase in the peripheral RBCs caused by a decrease of plasma volume, as with dehydration. *True (absolute) polycythemia* refers to an increase of total body hemoglobin–red cell mass. This may be secondary to an underlying disease or may be primary (idiopathic). When secondary to another disease state, "erythrocytosis" is probably a better term to apply, since it is usually associated with only increase of hemoglobin and red cell mass; about 98% of such cases result from decreased oxygen saturation of arterial blood, as with high altitude or disease of lungs or heart. *Primary polycythemia (rubra vera)* is a panmyelosis with abnormal proliferation of megakaryocytes, granulocytic and erythroid cells in the marrow, and increased numbers of all three cell types in the peripheral blood. Arterial oxygen saturation is normal, and there is no increased amount of erythropoietin in the blood.

■ **What is Di Guglielmo's disease?**

This refers to a "pure" erythroblastic malignant proliferation. There are bizarre megaloblastoid cells in the marrow and many nucleated RBCs in the peripheral blood (usually over 10 per 100 WBCs). *Di Guglielmo's syndrome* refers to a malignant erythroblastic proliferation combined with malignant proliferation of another cell type (e.g., myeloid: erythroleukemia).

■ **What is a likely diagnosis in a patient having 1.4 million RBCs, 4.8 gm hemoglobin, 3,800 WBCs, 14,000 platelets, and a reticulocyte count of 0.5%?**

The most likely diagnosis is a macrocytic anemia associated with megaloblastic dyspoiesis of the bone marrow and decreased numbers of all three cellular elements in the peripheral blood. Most often this is associated with pernicious anemia or a folic acid deficiency state.

■ **What are some of the likely diagnoses in a patient having a normocytic, normochromic anemia and an elevated platelet count?**

The most probable include acute blood loss and malignancy.

■ **In what condition may the mean corpuscular hemoglobin concentration go above the normal value?**

In hereditary spherocytosis; unlike mean corpuscular hemoglobin, MCHC is not increased in pernicious anemia.

The leukocytes

ALFRED MEYERS

■ **List and describe the usual WBC types seen in the peripheral blood.**

There are five different leukocyte types: neutrophilic granulocytes, eosinophilic granulocytes, basophilic granulocytes, monocytes, and lymphocytes. The granulocytes usually have a segmented or lobed nucleus; these lobes communicate by threads or filaments of nuclear membrane, which do not enclose obvious chromatin. A few less mature forms have a band- (or stab-) shaped nucleus. Neutrophilic bands are enumerated in the routine differential count and compose about 5% or less of the neutrophils. Lymphocytes can be divided into small and large subtypes. The former compose about 70% of the lymphocytes. (Your description should be compared with the detailed morphology of these cell types, which can be found in standard atlases of morphology.)

■ **Where are these cell types formed?**

The granulocytes (the neutrophils, eosinophils, and basophils) develop in the bone marrow. Monocytes also develop in the bone marrow. Lymphocytes originate from lymphoid tissue, which is widely distributed throughout the body.

Lymphoid tissue is found in the lining of the gastrointestinal tract, respiratory tract, and oropharynx. The oropharynx contains the tonsils and adenoids. These lymphoid sites are continually exposed to and stimulated by foreign antigen. Lymph nodes are situated strategically at many points in the connective tissue of the body and represent drainage stations for lymphatic vessels. These lymphatics will transport foreign antigen (macrophage-borne) or "messenger" lymphocytes away from local tissue sites of injury. These cells can stimulate nodal lymphoid proliferation, which will result in migration of lymphocytes into efferent lymphatics. The spleen is a major blood-filtering organ and has abundant lymphoid tissue, which is responsive to blood-borne antigen. Bone marrow also contains lymphocytes.

Lymphocytes continually recirculate. They leave the small blood vessels and, directly or indirectly, reenter the lymphoid tissues from which they or later generations of lymphocytes eventually will exit by penetrating the lymphatic sinuses, which drain into efferent lymphatics. The efferent lymphatics eventually empty into major veins and thereby start the recirculating process.

■ **Discuss the embryologic origin of lymphocytes.**

The embryologic origin of the small and large lymphocytes differs. The thymus is a lymphoid-rich organ responsible for colonizing lymphoid tissues with the progenitors of the small lymphs called T-lymphocytes. In childhood, the thymus is a prominent organ in the upper anterior chest, but it involutes markedly by early adulthood. The embryonic bone marrow and fetal liver contain lymphoid progenitors. They colonize developing adult lymphoid tissue with large lymphs called B-lymphocytes. Mature lymphoid tissue contains cells from these dual origins; moreover, they are arranged in compartments or domains that are architecturally fairly distinct. These embryologic and morphologic differences anticipate functional differences.

■ **Describe the significance of the sheep red cell rosetting technique to identify T-lymphocytes.**

Although the lymphocytes are divided into two major morphologic and functional populations, the differences in size and nuclear-cytoplasmic features are too subtle for accurate differentiation by the usual peripheral smear examination.

T-lymphocytes have surface receptors that will adhere spontaneously to sheep RBCs, forming a flower petal–like arrangement of red cells around the lymphocyte—the E-rosette. This technique can give a reasonable estimate of the proportion and concentration of T-lymphocytes. B-lymphocytes have surface immunoglobulin, and some contain receptors for C_3. These characteristics may be useful in identifying these cells. About one half of the nonrosetting lymphs are B-lymphs. (Other minor populations exist that neither form spontaneous rosettes nor have surface marker immunoglobulin.)

T-lymphopenia may be seen in congenital disorders of the thymus. In malignancies such as Hodgkin's disease, the decline of T-cells indicates a poor prognosis. In chronic lymphocytic leukemia, which is almost always B-cell leukemia, there is a high proportion of nonlabelled cells and the concentration of T-lymphocytes remains about normal.

Other atypical or immature lymphoid leukemias have been characterized in part by the presence or absence of these and other markers.

■ **Discuss the function of each type and subtype of the leukocytes. Indicate the life span of each.**

The neutrophilic granulocyte is a phagocytic cell. The neutrophilic granules are microbicidal and rich in the protein lactoferrin. The less conspicuous fine azurophilic granules are rich in enzymes (e.g., lysozyme, peroxidase, and hydrolase). After phagocytosis, the granules empty into the phagocytic vacuole, which forms a phagolysosome. Digestion then takes place.

The specific function of the eosinophil is not clear. These cells are prominent in inflammations associated with allergy and in parasitic infestations. However, they are not an unusual component in other injury-inflammatory responses but are present in lesser numbers. The eosinophilic granule is rich in the enzyme arylsulfatase. It is believed that the function of arylsulfatase is to decelerate the inflammatory response by destroying certain inflammatory factors released from the basophil and its close cousin the tissue mast cell. One such factor is the slow-reacting substance of anaphylaxis (SRS-A).

The granules of the basophil are rich in histamine and heparin. Histamine has vasodilatory effects. Heparin prevents coagulation of plasma and tissue juices. Other factors are present in the basophil, such as SRS-A. These substances are necessary for an effective inflammatory response. IgE is bound to basophils (and its tissue counterpart, the mast cell). Reaction with its specific antigen (allergen) causes degranulation.

The neutrophil, eosinophil, and basophil are short-lived cells, probably surviving several days or less. Once leaving the circulation, they do not reenter. Activation of the neutrophil hastens its demise.

The monocyte, like the neutrophilic granulocyte, is primarily phagocytic. In the tissues, it transforms to a macrophage. It cleans up the debris of the neutrophilic encounters. It is a more effective phagocyte against larger foreign particles and certain neutrophilic-resistant microorganisms. It is important in antigen processing and digestion of antigen-antibody complexes. The cell has regenerative capacity and is apparently long-lived but probably does not reenter the circulation.

The granulocytes and monocytes are nonspecific leukocytic immunocytes. They are part of the body defense or immune mechanisms that do not respond in an accelerated fashion to previously experienced foreign antigen.

Lymphocytes confer specific immunity. Previous experience with foreign antigens results in enhanced activity even decades after the primary exposure. When appropriately stimulated, activated B-lymphocytes will transform to secretory plasma cells. These secrete specific immunoglobulins. The small (or T-) lymphocyte is a cell that participates in delayed hypersensitivity reactions and graft-rejection reactions and has certain tumoricidal properties as well as antimicrobial properties. In contrast to the B-lymphocytes, there is no macromolecular immunoglobulin secretion, and its response is designated as "cell mediated."

The T-lymphs have certain properties or factors that are probably related to polypeptide formation. These can be demonstrated to transfer immunity, to cause migratory inhibition of mononuclear cells, and to have cytotoxic properties. The T-lymphocyte readily responds to the stimulation of the mitogen phytohemagglutinin; the B-lymphocyte shows little or no response. The T-lymphocytes may include a subpopulation of cells that exert certain regulatory helper or repressor effects on B-cell responses.

Lymphocyte survival may be long-lived. Certainly there is recirculation of a substantial proportion of unstimulated cells. The transformed or reactive lymphocytes may have a reduced survival, particularly the B-lymphocyte. A subpopulation of long-lived or memory B- and T-lymphocytes would account for the anamnestic response.

■ **How may the white blood count and percent differential lead to erroneous interpretation?**

A report of the total leukocyte concentration and its differential by percent must be corrected to absolute concentration for each of the components. Errors in calculations and failure to remember normal absolute concentration may lead to improper identification of specific population shifts. Increases in the concentration of a cell type or types imply (ordinarily) a need for their specific cellular defenses (e.g., neutrophilic phagocytosis). Decreases also must be explained by consideration of such factors that may affect cell production, release, and survival. The following are *approximate* adult normal values that can be used to determine shifts in leukocyte populations:

Neutrophils	2,500-7,500	(with approximately 5% or less bands)
Eosinophils and basophils	50-500	(eos./basos., approximately 5:1)
Lymphocytes	1,000-4,000	(Ts/Bs, approximately 4:1)
Monocytes	60-600	

Example 1

WBC 20,000/mm³	Percent differential	Absolute concentration/mm³	Change
Neutrophils	70 (12 bands)	14,000	Moderate increase
Eos./Basos.	5	1,000	Slight increase
Lymphocytes	15	3,000	None
Monocytes	10	2,000	Moderate increase

Interpretation: Phagocytic activity increased, as may be seen with bacterial infection and myocardial infarction.

Example 2

WBC 20,000/mm³	Percent differential	Absolute concentration/mm³	Change
Neutrophils	20	4,000	None
Eos./Basos.	2	400	None
Lymphocytes	70	14,000	Marked increase
Monocytes	8	1,600	Mild increase

Interpretation: Lymphocytosis predominates with need for specific immunity, as may be seen with viral infections or certain bacterial infections such as whooping cough.

Example 3

WBC 2,500/mm³	Percent differential	Absolute concentration/mm³	Change
Neutrophils	20	500	Marked decrease
Eos./Basos.	8	200	None
Lymphocytes	70	1,750	None
Monocytes	2	50	Slight decrease

Interpretation: Lymphocytosis is relative and not absolute. Neutropenia predominates. This picture may be seen with bone marrow depression (decreased cell production) or severe hypersplenism (decreased neutrophilic survival and sequestration).

■ **Define inflammation and the role of the white blood count and differential in assessing inflammatory conditions.**

Inflammation is the host's cellular and humoral response to cellular and/or tissue injury. Injury may result from the effects of (1) ischemia, e.g., myocardial infarction; (2) microorganisms, e.g., bacterial pneumonia, infectious mononucleosis; (3) physical agents, e.g., burn trauma; (4) chemical agents, e.g., lead intoxication; (5) immunologic derangements, e.g., autoimmune thyroiditis, glomerulonephritis; or (6) malignancies.

The peripheral blood serves as a conduit for the circulating defensive cells, which are derived from the production centers (bone marrow and lymphoid tissue). Inflammation is present at the site of injury. A clue to the nature of the injury as well as its intensity may be reflected by change (or lack of change) in leukocytic concentration in the peripheral blood. Usually, changes are more dramatic with acute than with chronic disorders. In addition, the WBC count and differential are important means by which one may follow the progress of diseases. The white blood count and differential generally lack specificity and give only indirect evidence for potential diseases.

■ **Indicate the neutrophilic changes often noted in acute inflammation.**

These changes may be listed as follows:

1. A substantial increase in neutrophilic concentration

2. A significant percentage increase in band forms and occasionally in less mature forms (a shift to the left)
3. Prominent azurophilic granulation (toxic granulation)
4. Döhle's bodies (cytoplasmic RNA)
5. Cytoplasmic vacuoles
6. Degranulation
7. Increased neutrophilic alkaline phosphatase content
8. Nuclear pyknosis

Not all these qualitative changes may be evident. Such changes are helpful in distinguishing the neutrophilic increases of emotional and physical stress from those of acute inflammation. An unfavorable prognosis may be anticipated if the neutrophilic response declines with an increasing proportion of bands and if the previously described cellular changes become increasingly pronounced.

■ **What is the Pelger-Huet anomaly? Indicate its significance.**

This autosomal dominant disorder is characterized by abnormal nuclear structure. The chromatin is overly condensed. The majority of neutrophils show decreased segmentation with peanut- or pince-nez–shaped nuclei resembling band forms. The heterozygotes have normal leukocytic function. If this anomaly is not recognized, a marked shift to the left may be reported and misinterpreted as severe acute inflammation.

■ **Analyze and discuss the following white blood count.**

A 30-year-old man with a palpable left neck mass.

WBC 12,000/*mm³*	*Percent differential*	*Absolute concentration/mm³*	*Change*
Neutrophils	30	3,600	None
Eos./Basos.	18/2	2,400	Marked increase
Lymphocytes	40	4,800	Slight increase
Monocytes	10	1,200	Slight increase

Eosinophilia predominates. Eosinophilia is accompanied usually by a slight increase of basophils. Mild eosinophilia may be seen in the healing phases of acute inflammation, such as following an operation. More intense eosinophilia is often noted with dermatitis, parasitic infestation, and many allergic disorders. In this case, because of a neck mass that may represent a lymph node tumor, one must consider a lymphoma, particularly Hodgkin's disease. Hodgkin's disease is frequently associated with pronounced eosinophilia, a reflection of the eosinophilic infiltrates in these nodes.

■ **Discuss the following white blood count in a febrile 16-year-old girl with deranged enzyme liver functions, in terms of practical clinical considerations and supportive morphologic alterations in leukocytes.**

WBC 15,000/mm³	Percent differential	Absolute concentration/mm³	Change
Neutrophils	44 (10% stabs)	6.600	Slight shift to left
Eos./Basos.	3	450	None
Lymphocytes	45	6,750	Moderate increase
Monocytes	8	1,200	Mild increase

The predominant change is lymphocytosis, which is commonly seen in acute viral infections and occasionally in certain specific non-viral infections. Autoimmune disorders may also show lymphocytosis. The prime consideration in this patient would be infectious mononucleosis with complicating hepatitis. A heterogeneous population of lymphocytes will be seen. Many are reactive or transforming stimulated lymphocytes—reactive cell-mediated T-lymphs and plasmacytoid B-lymphs. They exhibit cytoplasmic basophilia. Others are immature (proliferating) lymphs with large, irregular, light-staining nuclei. They may superficially resemble monocytes—hence the designation monocytoid lymphs. This impression of infectious mononucleosis should be confirmed by heterophile antibody study or EB virus titers. If these prove negative, one must consider other causes of the infectious mononuclear syndrome, such as infectious and serum hepatitis, cytomegalic inclusion disease, and toxoplasmosis.

■ **Discuss the clinical considerations when the only significant change in the white blood count and differential is absolute monocytosis.**

Mild monocytosis is seen in many clinical disorders, and although not to be ignored, it does not lead to specific considerations. When it is moderate or marked, i.e., threefold or more of the upper normal value, and unaccompanied by other significant shifts in leukocytic population, one should consider certain clinical disorders such as subacute bacterial endocarditis, disseminated tuberculosis, disseminated malignancy, and preleukemia and aleukemia.

■ **Define and discuss leukemoid reactions.**

A leukemoid reaction represents a peripheral blood picture that simulates leukemia. The leukocytosis may be profound, i.e., 50,000 or greater, with one cell type predominating and accompanied by a small but significant percentage of immature precursors of this cell type.

Neutrophilic leukemoid reactions generally show "toxic" changes (as outlined under neutrophilic changes often noted in acute inflammation). The alkaline phosphatase content of the neutrophils will be substantially elevated, in contrast to chronic granulocytic leukemia, in which it is usually depressed. Intense eosinophilia usually is reactive, and eosinophilic leukemia is rare. The primary underlying disorder should be identified. Marked intense basophilia is usually suggestive of a basophilic variant of chronic granulocytic leukemia. Lymphocytic leukemoid reactions usually result from infections such as infectious mononucleosis, infectious lymphocytosis, and whooping cough. If the cause is unsubstantiated by appropriate serologic and bacteriologic studies, bone marrow and lymph node examination may be necessary. Intense monocytosis or monocytic leukemoid reactions, although temptingly suggestive of monocytic leukemia, often prove to be nonleukemic and indicative of a severe systemic disease.

■ **What is the predominant change in the following white blood count? Discuss possible etiologic mechanisms.**

WBC 3,600/mm^3	Percent differential	Absolute concentration/mm^3	Change
Neutrophils	40	1,440	Moderate decrease
Eos./Basos.	5	180	None
Lymphocytes	45	1,620	None
Monocytes	10	360	None

There is moderate neutropenia. Initial considerations should be divided between causes of diminished leukopoiesis, abnormal cell release mechanisms, and decreased neutrophil survival or sequestration.

Decreased production may be caused by marrow injury. This may be seen with toxicity of overwhelming infection, drug and chemical toxicity, extensive irradiation damage, and extensive metastatic malignancy to bone marrow. Congenital leukopenia, which may be cyclic, represents a failure of myelopoiesis, the cause of which is uncertain. Depressed colony-stimulating factor (CSF) may be related to its pathogenesis. Subleukemia and preleukemia may occur with neutropenia as well as anemia and thrombopenia. Megaloblastic anemias usually have concomitant neutropenia and thrombocytopenia. The bone marrows are hypercellular and, although maturation is impaired, segmented neutrophils are readily evident.

The neutrophil will show decreased survival in severe infections, endotoxic shock, drug toxicity, and conditions in which autoimmune mechanisms are stimulated against neutrophils. Hypersplenism may be associated with significant sequestration of neutrophils as well as RBCs and platelets. Transient neutropenia is sometimes seen in the early stage of acute inflammation because of temporary depletion of circulating granulocytes. Neutropenias in blacks should not be confused with transient leukopenia. Blacks have a lower referent range than whites; this is usually not lower than 1,800 neutrophils, and marrow cellularity is normal.

■ **Define agranulocytosis and discuss possible etiologic mechanisms.**

In agranulocytosis there is complete absence of circulating granulocytes. This indicates either a profound destruction of circulating peripheral neutrophils or severe marrow damage with impairment of granulopoiesis. The disorder is usually discovered because of severe infection. Exposure to drugs and unusual chemicals or toxins must be determined. Many drugs have a bone marrow suppressive effect, which is manifested overtly with high dosages. A few patients may demonstrate a selective biochemical sensitivity or idiosynerasy to a drug with specific effects on dividing cells. In these patients, normal doses of such a drug will impair granulopoiesis. Occasionally drugs may induce an autoimmune reaction with the formation of leukoagglutinins. This may result in sudden, profound destruction of the circulating granulocytes.

■ **Discuss the granulocytic marginal pool and marrow reserve and possible tests for each.**

Increased numbers of mature granulocytes can be rapidly mobilized by physiologic stimuli such as exercise and anger. Their source is the marginal pool, which resides in the lung vasculature and to a lesser degree in the spleen. This resource can be tested by measuring granulocytic concentration before and after controlled epinephrine stimulation. Transient neutrophilia is not uncommonly seen in frightened children.

Bone marrow granulocytic reserve is a measure of the intensity and rapidity of cellular maturation and migration into the peripheral blood, the success of which is important in clinical infections. It can be studied by provocative testing with controlled stimulation of endotoxin, usually intravenously. The endotoxin may have an indirect stimulatory effect in that neutrophils activated by endotoxin may release CSF, which stimulates the marrow to hyperplasia, maturation, and release. Steroids may also be used as test substances.

■ **Discuss and comment on the following white blood count in a 3-year-old child with a history of many infections.**

WBC 5,000/mm³	Percent differential	Absolute concentration/mm³	Change
Neutrophils	75	3,750	None
Eos./Basos.	3	150	None
Lymphocytes	12	600	Marked decrease
Monocytes	10	500	None

A child normally has a higher absolute lymphocyte count than an adult. Therefore, this count indicates severe lymphopenia. This history suggests impaired immunity and probable diminished lymphopoiesis. Because the T-cells comprise about 70% of circulating lymphocytes, T-cell rather than B-cell depression is likely. This defect may be associated with thymic hypoplasia or aplasia and hypoplastic lymph nodes. Unless this is a combined defect, the globulin level should be normal. One could expect very little T-cell rosette formation. Skin testing for cell-bound immunity also should be impaired.

■ **Define and discuss balanced leukopenia.**

This is a decrease of neutrophils, lymphocytes, and, to a lesser extent, monocytes without significant alteration of their percentage differential. This combined depression could be expected when there is extensive damage to bone marrow and lymphoid tissue. This may be seen with drug therapy, e.g., cancer chemotherapy, and extensive irradiation. The disease process itself, e.g., malignancy, for which these modalities are often used, may involve the hemopoietic and lymphoid centers and further contribute to leukopenia. Another cause of balanced leukopenia is lupus erythematosus (LE), a systemic autoimmune disease with effects on leukocytes, erythrocytes, and platelets.

■ **Define and discuss pancytopenia.**

Pancytopenia is a decreased concentration of circulating leukocytes, erythrocytes, and platelets. This would indicate depressed myelopoiesis (myelo = marrow) or increased destruction or sequestration of all three elements. A few more common causes of impaired myelopoiesis are megaloblastic anemias, extensive irradiation, drug therapy with bone marrow depression, and extensive marrow infiltration with malignancy. Increased destruction of the circulating formed elements may be seen with severe infection, endotoxic shock, and autoimmune disorders such as LE. Hypersplenism may result in significant sequestration of all formed elements.

■ **Why are eosinopenia, basopenia, and monocytopenia given little recognition?**

The normal concentration of these cells is low, so that the differential may fail to reflect significant decreases. Moreover, when decreases are evident, concomitant changes in neutrophils or lymphocytes are more dramatic. Eosinopenia may be seen in hyperadrenalism (Cushing's disease). Monocytopenia is usually overshadowed by neutropenia.

■ **What is the Thorn test?**

This test determines the change of the absolute eosinophil count before and after ACTH stimulation. If there is a substantial drop in eosinophils to at least one-half the preinjection level, it is presumed that the adrenals are capable of secreting adequate corticoids. Adrenocorticoids cause eosinopenia and lymphopenia.

■ **Describe the LE cell and discuss the probable mechanism of its formation.**

The LE cell is usually a neutrophil that is distended by a large, relatively homogeneous, amphophilic mass slightly smaller than the neutrophil. This mass represents phagocytized, altered nuclear material that has interacted with autoimmune antinuclear antibodies and complement. The most significant nuclear antibody is that formed against native DNA. Neutrophils are chemotactic for complement and phagocytize the complex. In patients with LE, this phenomenon can be demonstrated with incubated peripheral blood, particularly when leukocytes are traumatized mildly by straining or whipping to allow exposure of antigenic nuclear material to the autoantibody. Extracellular altered nuclear masses surrounded by neutrophils, so-called rosettes, are often found in patients with LE but are not specific for this disorder. The LE cell is highly specific for LE, but the method is not sensitive. Occasionally, LE cells may be induced by certain antihypertensive drugs.

■ **What is a tart cell?**

This cell is usually a monocyte that has phagocytized nuclear material from damaged or dead cells. The engulfed mass retains basophilia and a nuclear chromatin pattern. Although common in LE, tart cells may be seen with other disorders.

■ **Describe other tests available to document antinuclear antibodies formed in LE.**

Indirect immunofluorescence has been the most popular screening test. It is quite sensitive and can be titered. Intact cells are used as a source of nuclear antigen, which can be supplied by tissues such as liver, by tissue culture cells, or by peripheral leukocytes from O-negative blood. Results will often be positive for other connective tissue disorders but not to the degree usually noted with untreated LE. Other serologic methods that demonstrate anti-DNA have been developed and include the latex agglutination test, precipitin immunodiffusion, and radioimmune assay. The efficacy of therapy will be manifested by decreasing titers of anti-DNA autoantibody. The disease activity is also correlated with complement levels that decline with increasing activity.

■ **Diagram the marrow evolution of primitive forms to granulocytes, erythrocytes, and platelets.**

°N, neutrophil; E, eosinophil; B, basophil; pmn, polymorphonuclear.

Small differences in terminology and in recognition and definition of cell categories may be noted in comparison to other schema. These differences are probably not of significant substance to detract from the usefulness of the outline, particularly in conceptualizing the myeloproliferative disorders.

■ **Define the myeloproliferative disorders.**

This is an abnormality of marrow tissue in which there is a seemingly *autonomous unrestrained proliferation* of myelopoietic cells. This usually involves one cell line of differentiation: granulocytic, erythrocytic, or megakaryocytic. Occasionally two or three cell lines are involved. Mature, intermediate, or primitive cells may predominate. Increased numbers of the overproduced cells, as well as lesser numbers of other immature cell forms, spill into the peripheral blood. If untreated, these disorders progressively worsen.

■ **Define and discuss chronic myelogenous leukemia.**

This is a myeloproliferative disorder in which there is marked granulopoiesis. The peripheral blood shows a substantial, often profound increase of mature granulocytes with a small percent of less mature forms. Although neutrophils generally predominate, basophils and eosinophils are also increased, and occasionally may predominate. Many of these leukemias show little or no alkaline phosphatase content within the cytoplasm of the neutrophil. Many also have a concomitant chromosomal abnormality with a translocation of the long arm of chromosome 22 (the Philadelphia chromosome). This can be demonstrated in the chromosomal structure of myeloid, erythroid, and megakaryocytic forms and supports the clonal nature of this disorder and of leukemia in general. These patients may live for several years until acute leukemic transformation or fatal infection occurs.

■ **Define and discuss acute myelogenous leukemia.**

This is a myeloproliferative disorder characterized by marrow hyperplasia and by peripheral blood dominated by immature precursors of the peripheral granulocytes. Myeloblasts, promyelocytes, or myelocytes may predominate. Anemia and thrombocytopenia are usual. No consistent chromosomal abnormality is evident. The clinical course of this group is usually very rapid, with the patient expiring because of hemorrhagic complications or infection.

■ **What is an Auer rod?**

This is an azurophilic, delicate, elongate crystalloid sometimes seen within the promyelocytes and monoblasts of leukemia cells. It represents an abnormal primary or azurophilic granule. Promyelocytic leukemia, in which Auer rods are prominent, is associated with more severe hemorrhagic complications and an associated element of consumptive coagulopathy.

■ **Define and discuss erythemic myelosis.**

This is an uncommon myeloproliferative disorder in which the marrow shows marked erythroblastic proliferation. The peripheral blood contains many erythroblasts. Proerythroblasts and basophilic erythroblasts predominate in acute erythemic myelosis; polychromatophilic and orthochromic erythroblasts predominate in chronic erythemic myelosis. These patients are anemic and often have atypical erythrocytes with megaloblastic forms. Acute erythemic myelosis has a rapidly fatal course. Polycythemia vera, which conceptually may be included in this classification, has the least pernicious prognosis.

■ **Define and discuss megakaryocytic myelosis.**

This is a rare myeloproliferative disorder characterized by excess proliferation of immature megakaryocytes. The cells are often atypical. There is severe thrombocytopenia, and megakaryocytic fragments are often seen within the peripheral blood. The disease is rapidly fatal. Primary thrombocythemia may be included conceptually in this classification and is characterized by hyperplasia of mature but atypical megakaryocytes. There is marked thrombocytosis, but these thrombocytes are functionally abnormal.

■ **Define and discuss myelofibrosis.**

Myelofibrosis is a myeloproliferative disorder characterized by patchy marrow fibrosis and interspersed panhyperplastic marrow. There is mild to moderate leukocytosis. The peripheral blood contains a small number of nucleated erythrocytes and immature myeloid elements. Platelets are usually increased in number and show variable size with large forms. The erythrocytes show considerable anisocytosis and poikilocytosis with characteristic teardrop forms. This disorder is often difficult to distinguish from chronic granulocytic leukemia. However, the leukocyte alkaline phosphatase is usually increased, and there is no associated Philadelphia chromosome. The marrow fibrosis is progressive, and intense extramedullary hemopoiesis occurs in the liver and spleen, which becomes greatly enlarged.

■ **List and discuss the mixed myeloproliferative disorders.**

Chronic granulocytic leukemia, polycythemia vera, idiopathic thrombocythemia, myelofibrosis, and erythroleukemia may be considered mixed myeloses. In early chronic granulocytic leukemia, polycythemia vera, and idiopathic thrombocythemia, the marrow generally shows hyperplasia of all three elements. Predominance of one of the three cell lines, however, usually characterizes the clinical course of the disorder. Polycythemia vera and idiopathic thrombocythemia may transform into chronic granulocytic leukemia or an acute myelosis. Myelofibrosis shows panhyperplasia accompanied by proliferation of stromal reticulum cells with marrow fibrosis and may terminate with blast transformation. The erythroleukemias show a mixed pattern. The peripheral blood and marrow show increases of immature myeloid and erythroblastic elements. This may eventually transform to a uniform acute myelosis. These overlapping patterns and transitions, sometimes associated with chromosomal changes in several cell lines, and the unity of enzymatic markers, which occur in heterozygotes, support the concept of an altered primitive cell as the clonal origin of these disorders.

■ **Define and discuss myelomonocytic leukemia.**

Both acute and chronic myelomonocytic leukemias may occur. Some are Philadelphia chromosome–positive and have diminished alkaline phosphatase content of neutrophils. Chronic myelomonocytic leukemia is a variant of chronic granulocytic leukemia. The peripheral blood contains mature granulocytes, an array of immature myelocytes, and a prominent monocytosis, i.e., 25%. The bone marrow is rich in immature myelocytes. Acute myelomonocytic leukemia has marrow and peripheral blood that are composed chiefly of immature myeloid elements and, in addition, primitive reticulohistiocytic cells. The reticulohistiocytic cells resemble monocytes.

■ **Define and discuss monocytic leukemia.**

Acute monocytic leukemia is a monoblastic leukemia. Its course is rapidly fatal. The monoblasts may contain Auer rods. Peripheral blood characterized by substantial increases of mature monocytes is most often a reactive rather than a leukemic condition. Therefore, marrow evaluation may be necessary.

■ **Define the lymphoproliferative disorders.**

This is an abnormality of lymphoid tissue in which there is a seemingly autonomous unrestrained proliferation of lymphopoietic cells. This involves one cell line of differentiation: T-lymphocytes or B-lymphocytes. The degree of differentiation may range from primitive precursors to well-differentiated cell-mediated lymphocytes or plasma cells, respectively. Usually the population is fairly homogeneous, but cellular atypia may occur. The overproduced cells often form solid tumors or may spill into the peripheral blood, presenting a leukemic picture, or they may have features of both. If untreated, these disorders become progressively worse.

■ **Define and discuss chronic lymphocytic leukemia.**

This is a lymphoproliferative disorder with marked mature lymphocytosis. Counts may be extremely high, i.e., 100,000 or more. It is accompanied by lymphocytic hyperplasia in lymphoid tissue. In the making of the peripheral smear, these lymphocytes are damaged easily and form smudge cells in and near the feather edge. The leukemic lymphocytes are clonal and almost always B-cells. Hypogammaglobulinemia or occasionally monoclonal gammopathy may develop. There is an increased association of autoimmune disorders, e.g., rheumatoid arthritis, and autoimmune hemolytic anemia may occur. Intense marrow involvement may compromise myelopoietic function. Although the clinical course is often protracted, life is usually shortened because of increased suspectibility to infection.

- **Define and discuss acute lymphocytic leukemia.**

This is a seemingly autonomous, unrestrained, progressive lymphocytosis in which the peripheral blood is dominated by lymphoblasts or prolymphocytes. In children, lymphoblastic leukemia is the most common leukemia. Prolymphocytic leukemia is seen in adults. Cell markers or absence of cell markers indicates differences in the lymphoid cell of origin of these leukemic cells. Although there are differences in clinical presentation, untreated disease is rapidly fatal and is associated with marrow replacement and complicating anemia, hemorrhage, and infection.

- **Discuss the differentiation of the acute leukemias and indicate pertinent cytochemical studies.**

The distinction between the acute lymphoblastic leukemias and the acute nonlymphoblastic leukemias is particularly important, because in children the former have had encouraging increases in length of survival and possible cures with specific programs of intensive chemotherapy. Characterization of blast forms sometimes may prove difficult with Romanowsky's stain. The different blast types sometimes show specific cytochemical reactions that aid in their differentiation. A small number of cases will fail to react with any of the special

Table 1. Cytochemical reactions of blast and pro forms in acute leukemia

	Acute lymphoblastic	*Acute granulocytic*	*Acute monocytic*
PAS	If present, a few (+) chunky particles	Usually (−), or diffuse faint (+) cytoplasmic tinge	Variable reaction: negative to heavy (+) coarse granules
Peroxidase	Uniformly (−)	Blasts: usually (−), or occasional (+) focal or faint reaction Pro form: (+)	Usually (−), or localized faint (+) cytoplasmic reaction
Sudan black B	Uniformly (−)	Strong *dense* localized (+) cytoplasmic activity	Discrete *scattered* (+) cytoplasmic granules
Esterase	Uniformly (−)	(+) Specific activity	(+) Nonspecific activity

stains. Several special stains should be used. The stains more commonly used include the PAS, peroxidase, sudan black, and esterase reactions. Lymphoblasts may show chunky PAS-positive granules in their cytoplasm; myeloblasts and monoblasts ordinarily do not. The peroxidase and sudan black reactions, although of different nature, give parallel results. They determine the presence of the primary or azurophilic granule. These may be seen in the immature myeloid forms. Myeloblasts usually do not react. Immature monocytes may give positive results, but their reactivity is more diffuse. Lymphoblasts do not have peroxidase activity. Esterase activity is reported to be most intense in the monocytic series.

■ **Define subleukemic and aleukemic leukemia.**

Subleukemic leukemia is that point in the clinical course of leukemia in which only a small number of leukemic leukocytes may be found within the peripheral blood. The marrow, however, will contain substantial numbers of leukemic cells adequate for diagnosis. In aleukemic leukemia the peripheral blood should contain no leukemic cells, but, as in subleukemia, the marrow will contain substantial numbers of leukemic cells. The peripheral blood may show mild leukocytosis, normal numbers of leukocytes, or leukopenia. Anemia and thrombocytopenia are often present. Monocytosis may be noted. It is the unexplained anemia, thrombocytopenia, leukopenia, or monocytosis that may be a clue to the possibility of leukemia. These definitions are applicable generally to acute leukemias, although in theory the chronic leukemias go through an aleukemia and subleukemia phase.

■ **Define and discuss preleukemia.**

This is a stage in the evolution of some leukemias in which there are no definitely recognizable changes within the peripheral blood and/or bone marrow. Hemopoietic abnormalities, when present, are not characteristic or of significant magnitude or specificity to make the diagnosis of leukemia. In preleukemic acute leukemia these changes include anemia, which may be megaloblastic, sideroblastic, or aplastic; leukopenia; thrombocytopenia; and unexplained monocytosis. Chromosomal studies may prove important, since a substantial proportion of these show abnormal karyotypes not unlike those seen in some of the acute leukemias. The preleukemic phase of the evolving chronic leukemia is often obvious in retrospect. It shows an insidious, slowly progressive leukocytosis of the cell type characteristic for that leukemia. If a chronic granulocytic leukemia is suspected, a chromosomal analysis for the Philadelphia chromosome may be diagnostic. The alkaline phosphatase content of the neutrophils may be significantly decreased in relation to the neutrophilia. Chronic lymphocytic leukemia will usually show disproportionate increases in B-lymphocytes.

■ **Define and discuss the lymphomas.**

The lymphomas are a group of solid tumor malignancies that involve the parenchymatous elements of lymphoid tissues. It includes those lymphoproliferative disorders that form solid tumors. Evidence indicates that the lymphoid lymphomas are clonal tumors of either T- or B-lymphocytes or their precursors, or are mature or transition forms of cell-mediated immunocytes and plasma cells. However, the lymphoma group also includes malignancies of the tissue histiocyte as well as the less defined malignancies of Hodgkin's disease and chronic leukemic reticuloendotheliosis (hairy-cell leukemia).

Generally, these malignancies initially form localized tumors that enlarge, invade surrouding tissues, and metastasize. The peripheral smear may give evidence of leukemic dissemination. This is not infrequent in lymphosarcomas. The leukemic lymphosarcoma cell usually shows significant morphologic atypia, such as folded and creased nuclei, and often can be distinguished from normal and leukemic lymphocytes. Some lymphosarcomas may be associated with dysproteinemia, monoclonal gammopathy, and hemolytic anemias. These are probably of B-cell origin.

Hodgkin's disease is a malignant lymphoma with a varied histologic pattern; often there is marked reactive inflammation and scarring. There are malignant cells interspersed in varying numbers. Their origin is uncertain. A characteristic and virtually diagnostic cell called the Reed-Sternberg cell is one of the major morphologic criteria of this disorder. The cell is a malignant bilobed multinucleated immunoblast. Eosinophilia is noted commonly with Hodgkin's disease. As the disease advances, immunity declines, particularly with reduction of T-cells and cell-bound immunologic phenomena.

In hairy-cell leukemia there are leukemic cells in addition to tissue involvement. The cell has delicate pointed cytoplasmic processes i.e., hairy processes. The exact nature of the cell is unclear. There is some morphologic resemblance to macrophages. Some cells have an immunoglobulin marker suggesting a B-cell relationship.

Table 2. Cytochemical and immunologic markers for lymphoid leukemias

	PAS°	Tartrate-resistant acid phosphatase	E-rosette†	Surface Ig
Lymphoblast	+	–	30%+	– or rare +
Mature T-lymphocyte	–	–	+	–
Mature B-lymphocyte	–	–	–	+
Lymphosarcoma T-cell	+	–	+	–
Lymphosarcoma B-cell	+	–	–	+
"Hairy cell"	–	+	–	–
Sézary cell	–	–	+	–

°(+) Applies to large, coarse granules or block of reactivity; only this type of particle is of diagnostic significance.
†Refers to percent of cases.

■ **List the lymphocytic and lymphocytoid leukemic cell types and discuss differential stains and surface markers helpful in their differentiation.**

Lymphoblasts and prolymphocytes, mature lymphocytes, lymphosarcoma lymphocytes, hairy-cell leukemic cells, and Sézary cells may not be significantly dissimilar in the peripheral smear with Romanowsky's stain to be identified with certainty. Several special stains and studies may be helpful. The stains more commonly used include the PAS and the acid phosphatase stain with and without tartrate inhibition. Determination of the presence or absence of a surface marker (i.e., E-rosette and immunoglobulin) is also helpful. Lymphoblasts often are PAS positive, but less than 30% will form E-rosettes; the remainder do not have any marker. Chronic lymphocytic leukemias ordinarily should cause no confusion, and most have a B-cell marker (immunoglobulin). Lymphosarcoma lymphocytes may have a B-cell marker or form E-rosettes. Leukemic hairy cells give positive results with the acid phosphatase stain, even after tartrate inhibition, which distinguishes them from other cells (Table 2).

■ **Define and discuss plasma cell myeloma.**

This is a malignant tumor of plasma cells that exhibits varying degrees of maturity and atypia. It usually involves the bone marrow, where there are localized and/or diffuse plasma cell infiltrates. Radiologic examination of the bone often shows characteristic punched-out lesions and/or osteoporosis. There may be hypercalcemia. Painful microfractures are common. Most myelomas are differentiated to the extent that there is secretion of excess immunoglobulin. The immunoglobulin is homogeneous, and a monoclonal pattern is evident in protein electrophoresis. IgG, IgM, IgA, and occasionally IgD and IgE may be synthesized. Excessive light-chain formation or inability to couple all the light with the heavy chains may result in light-chain secretion into the peripheral blood; sometimes only the light chain of the immunoglobulin molecule is synthesized. In either case, these light chains are filtered through the kidney into the urine as Bence Jones protein. Hyperglobulinemia will result in increased sedimentation rate and rouleaux formation in the peripheral blood smear. Atypical plasma globulins, e.g., cryoglobulins, may be formed. Anemia, which usually is present, may be aggravated by autoimmune anemia. As the disease progresses, the patients become increasingly susceptible to infection. Occasional cases terminate with plasma cell leukemia.

■ **Define and discuss Franklin's heavy-chain disease.**

This may be considered a variant of multiple myeloma in which the cells form and secrete a homogeneous heavy-chain fraction of the immunoglobulin molecules. The bone marrow will usually show a significant increase of plasma cells and lymphocytes. Lymphoid tissues show similar infiltrates. There is anemia and susceptibility to infection.

■ **Define and discuss Waldenström's macroglobulinemia.**

This is an unrestrained progressive proliferation of IgM secretory cells whose morphology is usually mixed, with B-lymphocytes, plasma cells, and intermediate or transitional cells between B-lymphocytes and plasma cells. The IgM is homogeneous and forms a monoclonal spike with protein electrophoresis. The infiltrates are noted in lymphoid tissue, but the bone marrow changes may not be as characteristic as in multiple myeloma. Bence Jones proteinemia is occasionally present. Rouleaux are prominent. Cryoglobulins may be noted. Minor hemorrhages are frequent, presumably due to interference of platelet function by the excessive concentration of IgM. These patients are anemic because of blood loss as well as decreased erythropoiesis; a hemolytic component may also be evident. There is increased susceptibility to infection. A leukemic picture may evolve.

■ **Define, discuss, and list causes of myelophthisic anemia.**

This is an anemia associated with marrow replacement and is sometimes called leukoerythroblastosis. It is associated with characteristic peripheral blood changes. There are small numbers of nucleated erythrocytes and immature myelocytes; the array of these cells is usually inclined to the more mature forms. Red cells show stippling, anisocytosis, and poikilocytosis with teardrop forms. Platelet concentration is variable, but more important, there is variability of size with giant forms. Extramedullary hemopoiesis or myeloid metaplasia may be present, particularly if the marrow involvement is extensive and the clinical course protracted. This occurs at sites that in the embryo were active in blood formation, e.g., spleen and liver.

Disorders that should be considered when the peripheral blood shows myelophthisic anemia include metastatic carcinomas, such as breast carcinoma; malignant lymphoreticular disorders, e.g., lymphosarcoma, multiple myeloma; myelofibrosis; histiocytoses of unknown etiology (Letterer-Siwe, eosinophilic granuloma); and certain lipid storage diseases with marrow infiltration by lipid-bearing cells.

■ **For each disorder listed, indicate briefly its significance and the cellular changes: Adler-Reilley anomaly; Chédiak's anomaly; May-Hegglin anomaly; vacuolated lymphocytes.**

The Alder-Reilley anomaly shows intense azurophilic granulation of granulocytes and occasionally of lymphocytes and monocytes. This may be seen alone or in association with hereditary disorders of mucopolysaccharide metabolism, one expression of which is gargoylism. In the mucopolysaccharidoses, one may also see lymphocytes with large purple inclusions within cytoplasmic vacuoles.

Chédiak's anomaly shows large, irregular azurophilic lysosomal granules in neutrophils. Eosinophilic and basophilic granules are abnormal as well. Lymphocytes and monocytes may contain azurophilic inclusions. This anomaly is associated with a defect in melanin production and with albinism. Leukopenia and thrombocytopenia are present. Infections are common and prove fatal in childhood.

The May-Hegglin anomaly shows coarse Döhle bodies in granulocytes, monocytes, and lymphocytes. Mild leukopenia is present. Giant platelets are present, and there may be thrombocytopenia. It is an autosomal dominant disorder whose major problem is associated with thromobocytopenia.

Vacuolated lymphocytes may be seen in several disorders. These include juvenile amaurotic idiocy (Tay-Sachs disease), which is a lipidosis associated with abnormal ganglioside metabolism; Niemann-Pick disease, another lipidosis, caused by sphingomyelin accumulation; and glycogen storage disease.

■ **For each disorder listed, indicate briefly its significance and the cellular changes: Niemann-Pick disease and Gaucher's disease.**

Niemann-Pick disease is a disorder of sphingomyelin metabolism caused by an abnormality of sphingomyelinase. Large macrophages with abundant foamy cytoplasm form because of the accumulation of sphingomyelin and sterols. The disease is found in children and is associated with mental and physical retardation. Death usually occurs early because of infection.

Gaucher's disease is a disorder of lipid metabolism caused by an abnormality of beta-glycosidase. There is accumulation of cerebroside within macrophages, forming large cells with a striate appearance. The disease may occur in children or adults. In children there is mental retardation.

In both of these disorders, diagnosis may be made presumptively by the characteristic appearances of these lipid-filled cells. The bone marrow is a convenient source of demonstrating these cells.

■ **Discuss the possible cause of chronic granulomatous disease and the nitroblue tetrazolium (NBT) test.**

This disease is an example of abnormal neutrophilic function without morphologic expression. These patients have recurrent infection, possibly caused by a group of closely related enzymatic disorders, some of which may be sex-linked and occur in males. Phagocytosis is not impaired, but there is selective loss of bactericidal activity. The enzymatic defect in the neutrophil is apparently caused by diminished effectiveness or formation of peroxide, which is reduced to sublethal levels by catalase-producing organisms. *Staphylococcus aureus, Serratia,* and *Candida* infections are common. This selectivity is apparently a result of catalase activity that is protective of these organisms. In non–catalase producers such as the streptococci, the neutrophil has adequate bactericidal activity.

This defect can be demonstrated by inducing a burst of oxidative activity. Stimulated granulocytes will reduce NADH. The reduced NADH will interact with the NBT dye, forming a blue formazan compound. NADH reduction is impaired in this disorder, and therefore, production of the blue formazan dye is reduced. This reaction can be quantitated by supernatant studies or by scoring the granulocytes.

CHAPTER 3

Immunohematology

Gordon E. Lang

■ **List twenty historical landmarks that have been important to the field of immunohematology.**

1616 William Harvey discovered the circulation of blood.

1656 Sir Christopher Wren injected various medications into the veins of dogs.

1665 Richard Lower performed the first successful transfusion from the carotid artery of one dog into the jugular vein of another dog.

1667 Jean Baptiste Denis performed the first recorded transfusion of a human. Lamb blood was given to a young man.

1818 James Blundell performed the first transfusion of human blood to another human.

1901 Karl Landsteiner discovered ABO blood groups.

1914 L. Agote administered the first transfusion of human blood that utilized sodium citrate as an anticoagulant.

1916 Rous and Turner demonstrated that the addition of dextrose to citrated blood exerted a favorable effect on the preservation of blood.

1937 Fantus opened the first blood bank in the United States. It was located in Chicago at Cook County Hospital.

1940 Landsteiner and Weiner reported the Rh blood factor.

1943 Loutit and Mollison described the use of ACD (acid-citrate-dextrose) solution for the preservation of blood.

1945 Coombs, Mourant, and Race described the use of the anti–human globulin test, which was based on the observations of Moreschi (1908), for the detection of "incomplete" Rh agglutinins.

1950 Audrey Smith demonstrated that erythrocytes mixed with glycerol could be frozen and thawed without injury.

1952   Jean Dausset described the occurrence of leukocyte isoantibodies in the serum of patients transfused with blood from many donors. This led to the development and understanding of the HLA system in relation to survival of organ transplants.

1953 and 1954   Valtis and Kennedy reported that a marked shift to the left (decreased P_{50}) occurred in the oxygen-hemoglobin dissociation curve when blood was stored for a week or more in the ACD solution.

1957   Gibson and associates described the use of CPD (citrate-phosphate-dextrose) solution for the preservation of blood.

1958   Dudley and associates described the use of plastic bags for storing and transfusing blood.

1961   Stern first reported that passive administration of anti-Rh_0 (**D**) would prevent primary Rh immunization.

1965   Blumberg and associates described the occurrence of the Australia antigen (hepatitis-associated antigen) in patients with hepatitis.

1967   Benesch and Benesch and Chanutin and Curnish independently reported that the shift to the left in the O_2 dissociation curve (decreased P_{50}) that occurs in ACD-stored blood resulted from a decreasing concentration of 2,3-diphosphoglycerate (2,3-DPG).

■ **What is an antigen?**

An antigen is any substance (usually protein in nature) that, when introduced into an individual who himself lacks the substance, stimulates the production of an antibody and that, when mixed with the specific antibody, reacts with it in some observable way, such as agglutination, hemolysis, or precipitation.

■ **What is an antibody?**

An antibody is a specific substance (usually a globulin) produced by an individual in response to the introduction of an antigen. The antibody will react specifically with that antigen in some observable way, as described above.

■ **What are hemagglutinogens, hemagglutinins, and isohemaglutinins?**

Antigens present on the surface of erythrocytes are referred to as hemagglutinogens, and antibodies that agglutinate erythrocytes are referred to as hemagglutinins. Isohemagglutinins are antibodies that agglutinate erythrocytes of another member of the same species.

■ **What is isoimmunization?**

Isoimmunization is the formation of immune antibodies by a member of a given species against some antigen normally absent from its own body but present in another member of the same species. Rh_0 (D)–positive blood transfused to an Rh_0 (D)–negative individual can result in isoimmunization to the Rh_0 (D) isoagglutinogen.

■ **What is a hemolysin?**

A hemolysin is a type of antibody that, in the presence of complement, results in liberation of hemoglobin from the erythrocytes.

■ **What is complement?**

Complement consists of a series of nine plasma components that react sequentially and are necessary to produce hemolysis. According to the World Health Organization nomenclature and reaction sequence, they are C1, C4, C2, C3, C5, C6, C7, C8, and C9. C1 is composed of three subcomponents: C1q, C1r, and C1s. Intermediate complexes formed by the reaction of the erythrocyte and the antibody with the various components are named according to the complement-component bond. Calcium and magnesium are required for completion of the reaction sequence, and therefore, anticoagulants that bind these cations inhibit complement-dependent reactions. Heating serum to 56° C for 30 minutes completely inactivates C1 and C2 and partially inactivates C4.

■ **What is agglutination?**

Agglutination is the visible clumping reaction that occurs when suspensions of erythrocytes, latex particles, or bacteria containing specific antigens are mixed with a serum containing specific antibodies for those antigens.

■ **What is the ABO blood group system? Indicate the major groups within this sytem.**

The ABO blood group system was the first human blood group system discovered. Landsteiner in 1901 found that human blood could be classified into three groups—A, B, and O. One year later Landsteiner's students, Decastello and Sturli, discovered the group AB. The ABO classification is based on the presence of either, neither, or both of two antigenic and type-specific polysaccharide substances, A and B, on the surface of the erythrocyte. The groups are named for the antigen (agglutinogen) present on the erythrocyte.

Antigen present	Blood group
A	A
B	B
A and B	AB
Neither	O

■ **What is a major difference between the ABO blood group system and the other blood group systems?**

The ABO blood group system is the only system that regularly contains "naturally occurring" antibodies (agglutinins) within serum. These agglutinins do not react with the erythrocytes that are suspended in the serum. All of the other blood group systems do not regularly have "naturally occurring" antibodies in the serum. In other systems, antibodies develop secondary to artificial immunization following blood transfusion or pregnancy. The "naturally occurring" antibodies (agglutinins) of the ABO blood group system are:

Blood group	Antibody present
A	Anti-**B**
B	Anti-**A**
AB	Neither
O	Anti-**A** and anti-**B**

■ **Discuss the cross-reacting anti-A, B (C) present in group O serum.**

It is well-known that absorption of group O serum with either A or B erythrocytes will reduce the titer of both anti-**A** and anti-**B**. This finding led to the discovery that group O serum contains—in addition to anti-**A**, anti-**A**$_1$, and anti-**B**—anti-**A**, **B** (**C**). Group O serum reacts with all of the various subgroups of A and all B erythrocytes but does not react with O cells. Group O serum must be used to prove that erythrocytes reacting negatively to anti-**A** and anti-**B** serum are truly O cells. Certain rare cells that are not O cells (e.g., A$_x$) will react negatively with anti-**A** and anti-**B** serum as do O cells. However, when these cells are reacted with group O serum, agglutination occurs. This reaction is caused by the presence of anti-**A**, **B** (**C**) in the group O serum. It is believed by most investigators that anti-**A**, **B** reacts with a portion of the A or B antigen that is in common and therefore cross-reacts. Others have proposed the presence of another antigen (**C**).

■ **What is absorbed B or anti-A₁ serum?**

A$_1$ erythrocytes can be easily separated from A$_2$ erythrocytes by reacting them with group B serum that has been absorbed with A$_2$ erythrocytes. This absorption removes anti-**A**, which reacts with both A$_1$ and A$_2$ cells, but does not remove anti-**A**$_1$, which reacts only with A$_1$ erythrocytes. Therefore, absorbed B serum will react only with A$_1$ erythrocytes.

■ **What are the subgroups of A?**

In 1911 it was discovered by von Dungern and Hirszfeld that there were subgroups of A or variants of antigen A. Anti-A serum obtained from group B individuals contains two isoagglutinins: anti-**A**, which reacts with all group A and AB erythrocytes, and another isoagglutinin, anti-A_1, which reacts in only about 80% of individuals with group A or AB erythrocytes. Individuals who react with anti-A_1 are called A_1, and those who do not are called A_2.

The practical importance of the A subgroups (A_1, A_2, A_1B, and A_2B) is that A_2 and especially A_2B erythrocytes may react more weakly with anti-A serum than do A_1 and A_1B erythrocytes, and their detection may be missed. It is also important that about 1% of A_2 individuals and 25% of A_2B individuals have anti-A_1 in their plasma. These individuals cannot be transfused with blood that contains the A_1 antigen.

Several other subgroups have been described, namely A_3, A_m, and A_x. These cells generally react weakly or not at all with group B serum. They are all agglutinated by serum from group O individuals. When reacted with group B serum, A_3 erythrocytes agglutinate in a mixed field pattern, i.e., some cells agglutinate and others do not. A_m cells may react negatively with group O and group B serum. A and H substances are present in the secretions (saliva, etc.) of these individuals if they are secretors. The reactions of the subgroups are summarized at the top of p. 47.

- **What are agglutinins obtained from plants called?**

Lectins are extracts obtained from certain plants that agglutinate red cells of a particular antigen. Examples are:

Plant	Agglutinin present
Dolichos biflorus	anti-A_1
Ulex europaeus	anti-**H**
Iberis amara	anti-**M**
Vicia graminea	anti-**N**
Bandeiraea simplicifolia	anti-**B**
Arachis hypogoea (peanut)	anti-**T**

Extracts from some snails have anti-**A** activity.

- **What is H substance? What happens when the gene responsible for H substance is absent?**

Most human erythrocytes contain a basic substance called H substance. This substance, under the influence of the *A* or *B* gene located on chromosome 9, is converted to A or B substance. O erythrocytes contain the largest quantity of H substance and AB the least. The reaction strength of anti-**H** with various blood groups in descending order is $O > A_2 > A_2B > B > A_1 > A_1B$. Anti-**H** may be found in the plasma of a rare A_1, A_1B, or B individual whose erythrocytes contain very little H substance.

	Direct grouping						Reverse grouping (cells)			
Pheno-type	Anti-A group B serum	Anti-B group A serum	Anti-A₁ absorbed B serum	Lectin Dolichos biflorus	Anti-A, B (C)	Anti-H	A₁	A₂	B	O
A_1	+	−	+	+	+	±	−	−	+	−
A_2	+	−	−	−	+	+	−	−	+	−
A_3	+mf°	−	−	−	+mf°	+	−	−	+	−
A_x (A_4)	−or±	−	−	−	+	+ or +	−	−	+	−
A_m	− to vwk°	−	−	−	−to vwk°	+	−	−	+	−

°mf, mixed field; vwk, very weak.

A very rare individual contains no H, A, or B substance on his erythrocytes. The plasma of this individual contains anti-H, anti-A, and anti-B. The blood group of this individual is called Bombay or Oh. He lacks an *H* gene, which normally converts a basic precursor substance to H substance, which in turn is acted on by *A* and/or *B* genes to form A and B substance.

Normal: Precursor substance $\xrightarrow{H \text{ gene}}$ H $\xrightarrow[B \text{ gene}]{A \text{ gene}}$ A   B

Bombay: Precursor substance $\longrightarrow$ □ $\xrightarrow[B \text{ gene}]{A \text{ gene}}$ □

The reactions of group O and group Oh individuals with known anti-sera and cells are summarized below.

Bombay individuals will transmit to their children *A* and/or *B* genes if they possess them. Mating between an Oh and an O individual could result in an A or B child.

■ **Compare the immunoglobulins.**

Immunoglobulins are specific proteins produced by plasma cells that are formed from B-lymphocytes following antigenic stimulation. Five distinct classes of immunoglobulins have been described: IgA,

	Direct grouping						Reverse grouping (cells)			
Pheno-type	Anti-A group B serum	Anti-B group A serum	Anti-A₁ absorbed B serum	Lectin Dolichos biflorus	Anti-A, B (C)	Anti-H	A₁	A₂	B	O
O	−	−	−	−	−	+	+	+	+	−
Oh	−	−	−	−	−	−	+	+	+	+

IgG, IgM, IgD, and IgE. The blood group antibodies are associated with the IgA, IgG, and IgM classes.

The basic immunoglobulin molecule consists of two heavy polypeptide chains and two light polypeptide chains. The heavy chains are connected to each other by a disulfide bond (—S—S—); a light chain is connected to each heavy chain by a similar bond (—S—S—).

The heavy chains are specific for each class of immunoglobulin, whereas the light chains of the five classes have similar characteristics and have been designated as kappa and lambda. The IgG class has been divided into four subclasses, the IgA into two subclasses.

The immunoglobulins that are produced following initial exposure to a foreign antigen are usually of IgM specificity, whereas during subsequent exposure IgG is produced. Table 3 summarizes the immunoglobulins.

■ What are Fab and Fc?

The enzyme papain splits the IgG molecule into three fragments. Two of the fragments are identical and are named Fab (fragment antigen binding). They are composed of a light chain and part of a heavy

Table 3. Immunoglobulin characteristics

	IgG	*IgA*	*IgM*	*IgD*	*IgE*
Molecular weight	150,000	150,000	1,000,000	150,000	190,000
Sedimentation constant	7S	7S-18S	19S	7S	8S
Concentration, mg/dl (average)					
Adult	1,200	300	100	2	0.03
Cord blood	600	0	10	–	–
Placental transfer	Yes	No	No	No	No
Length	250A		1,000A		
Gm allotype	Yes	No	No	No	No
Inv allotype	Yes	Yes	Yes	Yes	Yes
Erythrocyte agglutination activity	Incomplete	Incomplete	Complete	None	None
Heavy chains	Gamma (γ)	Alpha (α)	Mu (μ)	Delta (δ)	Epsilon (ϵ)
Light chains	Kappa (κ), lambda (λ)	κ, λ	κ, λ	κ, λ	κ, λ
Molecular formula	$\gamma_2\kappa_2$, $\gamma_2\lambda_2$	$(\alpha_2\kappa_2)_{1-3}$ $(\alpha_2\lambda_2)_{1-3}$	$(\mu_2\kappa_2)_5$ $(\mu_2\lambda_2)_5$	$\delta_2\kappa_2$ $\delta_2\lambda_2$	$\epsilon_2\kappa_2$ $\epsilon_2\lambda_2$
Subclasses	$\gamma_{1,2,3,4}$	$\alpha_{1,2}$	$\mu_{1,2}$	–	–
Complement fixation	$\gamma_{1,2,3}$ yes; γ_4 no	No	Yes	No	No

chain. The third fragment, termed Fc (fragment crystalline), is composed of part of two heavy chains. Fab fragments contain the antigen-combining sites, and the Fc fragment is responsible for complement fixation, placental transportation, skin sensitization, and other functions.

■ **Discuss the development of the isoagglutinins of ABO system.**

At birth about 40% of infants have no detectable isoagglutinins in their serum. In the remaining 60% of infants, the isoagglutinins are passively transferred from the mother and isoagglutinin is produced by the infant. The passively transferred isoagglutinin has IgG specificity, whereas the isoagglutinin produced by the infant before birth has IgM specificity. Significant levels of the ABO isoagglutinins are detected between 3 and 6 months of age; the maximum titer is attained at 5 to 10 years of age. The ABO isoagglutinins have traditionally been divided into two types: the "naturally occurring" and the "immune occurring" isoagglutinins. The naturally occurring isoagglutinins are thought to be produced as an immune response to ingested or inhaled antigenic substances found in nature that are similar to human A and B substances. The immune occurring isoagglutinins are found in persons who have been stimulated with A and B substances following incompatible transfusions, heterospecific pregnancies (e.g., O mother, A child), or injections of soluble blood group substances or other materials such as vaccines, which may contain A and/or B substances. The characteristics of the naturally occurring anti-A and the immune anti-A isoagglutinins are outlined in Table 4.

■ **Discuss the inheritance of the ABO blood group system.**

The ABO blood group of an individual is determined by the genes that he inherits from his parents.

Table 4. Comparison of naturally occurring and immune anti-A

	Natural	Immune
Reacts with saline-suspended cells	Yes	No
Antihuman globulin test required to detect	No	Yes
Neutralized by soluble blood group substances (Witebsky substances)	Yes	No
Lyses erythrocytes	Few	Most
Binds complement	Yes	Only IgG, not IgA
Type of immunoglobulin	IgM	IgG or IgA
Heat	Labile	Stable
Reacts with pig A^p cells	No	Yes
Optimal temperature for reaction	Room temp.	37° C

Three allelic genes are responsible for the determination of the ABO genotype. The genes, ignoring the subgroups, are A, B, and O. The A and B genes give rise to the antigens A and B by converting H substance to A or B agglutinogen. The O gene is an amorph (a gene that does not produce any recognizable effect). It does not have any effect on H substance.

Each individual inherits one A, B, or O gene from each of his parents. Because the O gene is an amorph and recessive, it is only detectable in individuals who inherit it from both parents. Individuals who inherit only one O gene are phenotypically similar to individuals who are homozygous for either the A or the B gene (i.e., AA, AO; BB, BO).

With rare exceptions, the following rules have been applied to the inheritance of the ABO and other blood group agglutinogens.

1. An agglutinogen cannot be present in the blood of an individual unless it is present in the blood of one or both parents.
2. An individual who is homozygous for an agglutinogen must transmit the gene responsible to all of his children.
3. A child who is homozygous for an agglutinogen must have inherited the gene responsible from both of his parents.

Applying these statements to the ABO group, one can state that:

1. Agglutinogens A and B cannot be present in the blood of a child unless present in the blood of one or both parents.
2. A group AB parent cannot have a group O child.
3. A group O parent cannot have a group AB child.

■ **Indicate the ABO phenotypes of children that are possible if the ABO phenotypes of the parents are known.**

Phenotype of parents	Possible phenotypes of children
O + O	O
O + A	A or O
O + B	B or O
A + A	A or O
A + B	A or B or O or AB
B + B	B or O
O + AB	A or B
A + AB	A or B or AB
B + AB	A or B or AB
AB + AB	A or B or AB

■ **What is meant by secretor or nonsecretor status of an individual?**
About 80% of white individuals contain H substance in their saliva

and other body fluids. These individuals, if they are also group A, B, or AB, will also have A or B substance in their saliva. The remaining 20% of white individuals are known as nonsecretors—these substances are not present in their saliva or other body fluids. The secretor status is inherited as a mendelian dominant trait. The gene responsible for secretor status is called *Se* (allele *se*). Secretors may be of genotype *SeSe* or *Sese*, whereas nonsecretors are of the genotype *sese*.

The A, B, and H substances in body fluids are water soluble. The A, B, and H substances in erythrocytes and other tissues are alcohol soluble, and their presence is not determined by the secretor gene.

The *Se* gene interacts with the Lewis gene *(Le)* so that most secretors of ABH substances are Lewis (Le^a) negative, and most nonsecretors of ABH substances are Lewis (Le^a) positive.

■ **How does the Lewis blood group system differ from the other blood group systems?**

The antigens of all blood group systems except the Lewis system are an integral part of the red cell membranes. The Lewis antigens are water-soluble plasma and salivary antigens that are absorbed onto the surface of the membranes of erythrocytes. Cord blood is generally nonreactive or only very weakly reactive to anti-**Le**^{a} or anti-**Le**^{b}. Lewis reactivity is not apparent until the infant is several weeks old, at which time the concentration of plasma Lewis substance is adequate for red cell absorption. The Lewis genes are designated as *Le* and *le*. The production of Le^a substance is controlled by the *Le* gene, which is dominant. The *le* gene is an amorph. Le^b substance results from the conversion of Le^a substances under the influence of the *H* and *Se* gene. The A, B, H, and Lewis substances are derived from the same precursor. The interrelationship of the ABO, Lewis, and secretor status can best be briefly explained by Table 5.

The table reveals that individuals in the phenotype Le(a+b−) are nonsecretors of A, B, or H substances. Individuals who are *Se* positive, *Le* positive generally produce insufficient Le^a substance to result in erythrocytes that are Le^a positive and are thus of the phenotype Le(a−b+). Rare O or A$_2$ individuals may not convert all of the Le^a substance to Le^b substance and thus may have the rare phenotype of Le(a+b+). On the other hand, *Se* positive, *Le* positive individuals of blood group A or B may have erythrocytes that react weakly with anti-**Le**^{b} because most of the Le^b substance has been converted to A or B substance.

Le^a substance is not converted to Le^b substance unless an indi-

Table 5. Schematic diagram of the ABO, Lewis, and secretor interrelationships

Substances in saliva	Lewis phenotype RBCs	Incidence Whites	Incidence Blacks
ABH	Le(a−b−)	3%	17%
A, B, H, Le^a, Le^b	Le(a−b+)	74%	55%
Le^a	Le(a+b−)	23%	22%
—	Le(a−b−)	0.6%	6%

A, B, H, Le^a, and Le^b substances in body fluids are water soluble, and their presence is determined by the secretor gene.
A, B, and H substances in erythrocytes and other tissue are alcohol soluble, and their presence is not determined by the secretor gene.

vidual possesses both the *H* and the *Se* gene; therefore, *H*-negative (Bombay, Oh) individuals are either Le(a+b−) or Le(a−b−).

■ **Briefly describe the antibodies of the Lewis system.**

Lewis antibodies are produced by Le(a−b−) individuals without known antigenic stimulation. Lewis substances are thought to be ubiquitous. The antibodies of this system are IgM, and all have the ability to bind complement. Reactivity of most Lewis antibodies is best below room temperature, with some reacting at 37° C and with non−gamma antihuman globulin serum.

Several varieties of Lewis antibodies have been described. Anti-**Le^a**, the most common, is found in about 12% of Le(a−b−) individuals. All individuals with this antibody have at least one *Se* gene and therefore secrete ABH substance. There is a decreased incidence of the group O genotype in individuals with anti-**Le^a**. Anti-**Le^b** is at times found as a weak antibody in serums that contain potent anti-**Le^a**. Individuals who produce pure anti-**Le^a** are of the phenotype Le(a−b−) and do not possess any *Se* genes; therefore, they do not secrete ABH substances. Two types of anti-**Le^b** have been described: one, designated as anti-**Le^{bL}**, reacts with Le^b-positive cells of groups A, B, O, and AB; the other, designated as anti-**Le^{bH}**, reacts only with Le^b-positive cells of group O individuals. Several other antibodies have been described that react only with Le(a−b−) cells of various secretor status.

■ **Describe the two major theories of inheritance of the Rh blood group system.**

The Fisher-Race theory of inheritance suggests that there are three pairs of allomorphic genes: *C, c; D, d;* and *E, e*. Three of these genes are present, closely linked at separate loci, on each of a pair of chromosomes. It was proposed that each gene is responsible for producing antigenic material capable of stimulating agglutinins. To date, no antibodies to —d— have been identified.

The Weiner theory postulates that there are eight standard allelic genes, one gene located at a single locus on each of a pair of chromosomes. The Weiner genes are R^0, R^1, R^2, R^z, r, r', r'', r^y. Each of these genes is responsible for the production of complex antigens that have several different serologic specificities called factors. The correspond-

Table 6. Comparison of Weiner and Fisher-Race nomenclatures

Genes				Weiner antigens (8)	Weiner factors (6)		Fisher-Race antigens (6)	
Weiner (8)		Fisher-Race (6)						
		c			hr'	.80	c	.80
R^0	.027	D	.027	Rh_0	Rh_0	.85	D	.85
		e			hr"	.97	e	.97
		C			rh'	.70	C	.70
R^1	.41	D	.41	Rh_1	Rh_0	.85	D	.85
		e			hr"	.97	e	.97
		c			hr'	.80	c	.80
R^2	.15	D	.15	Rh_2	Rh_0	.85	D	.85
		E			rh"	.30	E	.30
		C			rh'	.70	C	.70
R^z	.002	D	.002	Rh_z	Rh_0	.85	D	.85
		E			rh"	.30	E	.30
		c			hr'	.80	c	.80
r	.38	d	.38	rh	Hr_0	.63	d	.63
		e			hr"	.97	e	.97
		C			rh'	.70	C	.70
r'	.006	d	.006	rh'	Hr_0	.63	d	.63
		e			hr"	.97	e	.97
		c			hr'	.80	c	.80
r''	.005	d	.005	rh"	Hr_0	.63	d	.63
		E			rh"	.30	E	.30
		C			rh'	.70	C	.70
r^y	.0001	d	.0001	rh^y	Hr_0	.63	d	.63
		E			rh"	.30	E	.30

ing Weiner genes, antigens, and factors and Fisher-Race genes and antigens are compared in Table 6. The Rh genes are located on chromosome 1.

R' ⟶ Weiner—one gene per chromosome

■ **Discuss the nomenclature of the Rh blood group system; include phenotypes, genotypes, and gene frequency.**

Two distinctly different nomenclatures have evolved: one is based on the Weiner theory of inheritance of the Rh antigenic determinants and the other on the Fisher-Race theory. Both nomenclatures are widely used, and the blood bank technologist must be familiar with both. Table 6 gives the corresponding equivalent terms for both nomenclatures. The numbers to the right of the genes, antigens, and factors are the frequencies of these in whites. These are used to calculate genotype frequency.

Phenotype is defined as the observable reaction or characteristics of an individual. The Rh phenotype is determined by observing the reactions of the five standard antisera: anti-**Rh$_0$** (D), anti-**rh'** (C), anti-**rh″** (E), anti-**hr'** (c), and anti-**hr″** (e). The Fisher-Race phenotype is written by observing cell reaction with these sera and first writing the Cs, then the Ds, and finally the Es to indicate the antigens present, e.g., CcDEe. The Weiner phenotype is more difficult, because it requires memorization of the Weiner antigens as determined by the reactions with the three Rh antisera and the two hr antisera, e.g., Rh$_0$rh (Fisher-Race phenotype ccDee). If the Rh$_0$ (D) factor is present, list the corresponding Weiner antigen first, e.g., Rh$_0$rh. Rh is only used when the Weiner Rh$_0$ (D) factor is included in the Weiner antigen. If the Rh$_0$ (D) factor is absent, the symbol rh is used. Subscripts 1, 2, and Z and superscripts ′, ″, and y are used to indicate the presence of the other blood factors rh′, rh″, and rh′rh″, e.g., Rh$_2$rh^y. Genotype refers to the genes possessed by an individual for a particular trait. The Fisher-Race Rh genotype can be estimated from the phenotype with some degree of accuracy by examining the phenotype and making sets of genes listing all possible combinations. Assign one set to the left and one set to the right of a slash mark, e.g., *CDe/cde*. If *D* is present in one set and not in the other, the set with the *D* should be to the left of the slash. The possible genotypes in an individual with phenotype CCDEe are *CDE/CDe, CDE/Cde,* and *CDe/CdE*.

The Weiner Rh-Hr genotype is determined by listing all of the Weiner gene combinations possible from inspection of the phenotype. In heterozygote Rh$_0$ individuals, the gene containing the Rh$_0$ factor should be given first, e.g., R^1r. The capital R indicates that the gene has the Rh$_0$ blood factor, and the lowercase r indicates that the Rh$_0$ blood factor is not present. Superscripts 1, 2, Z, ′, ″, and y are used to designate the presence of other blood factors, rh′, rh″, and rh′rh″. No subscripts and no *h*s are used in genotype designation. The possible genotypes in an individual of phenotype Rh$_z$Rh$_1$ (CCDEe) are R^ZR^1, $R^Zr′$, and R^1r^y.

The determination of the most probable genotype is important in the proper antenatal evaluation of possible hemolytic disease of the newborn. All children of a homozygous Rh_0 (D) father will have the Rh_0 factor, whereas only 50% of the children of a heterozygous Rh_0 (D) father and Rh_0 (D)–negative mother will have the factor.

The most probable genotype is determined by ascertaining the frequencies of the various genotypes. The genotype with the highest frequency is the most probable genotype. The calculation of genotype frequencies is simple. The frequency of a genotype with two like genes, e.g., *rr*, is the square of the gene frequency.

> Frequency of *r* gene is: 0.38
> ∴ Frequency of gentotype *rr* is: 0.38^2 or $0.38 \times 0.38 = 0.144$
> $0.144 \times 100 = 14.4\%$

The frequency of a genotype with two unlike genes is twice the product of the gene frequencies.

> Frequency of *r* gene is: 0.38
> Frequency of R^1 gene is: 0.41
> ∴ Frequency of genotype $R'r$ is: $2 \times 0.38 \times 0.41 = 0.312$
> $0.312 \times 100 = 31.2\%$

■ **What is the numerical system of designating the Rh-Hr blood group?**

A third method of identifying the Rh-Hr blood factors has been described by Rosenfield. Each Rh factor is designated by number. The phenotype Rh_2rh (ccDEe) would be written Rh: 1, −2, 3, 4, 5. The numbers corresponding to Weiner factors and Fisher-Race antigens are given in Table 7.

■ **What is the D^u ($\Re h_0$) variant?**

D^u ($\Re h_0$) is an Rh antigen that reacts weakly or not at all with the usual saline and/or slide anti-Rh_0 (D) sera. Those that react weakly are referred to as "high grade" D^u, and those that are nonreactive and require antihuman globulin sera for their detection are called "low grade" D^u.

Table 7. Comparison of Weiner, Fisher-Race, and Rosenfield nomenclatures

Weiner factor	Fisher-Race antigen	Rosenfield number
Rh_0	D	Rh_1
rh'	C	Rh_2
rh"	E	Rh_3
hr'	c	Rh_4
hr"	e	Rh_5

Some of the so-called high-grade D^us result from a gene interaction effect exerted by the presence of the r' *(Cde)* gene on the gene on the opposite chromosome, which determines Rh_0 (D). This gene interaction results in a suppressed reactivity of the Rh_0 (D) antigen.

The remaining high-grade and low-grade D^us ($\mathfrak{R}h_0$) are genetically weak antigens that are passed from one generation to another. According to the Weiner theory, the Rh_0 (D) factor is composed of four components, Rh^A, Rh^B, Rh^C, and Rh^D. The lack of one or more of these components results in a weak-reacting $\mathfrak{R}h_0$ variant, the so-called D^u ($\mathfrak{R}h_0$).

■ **What is the G antigen of the Rh system and what is its significance?**

The G, rh^G, or Rh_{12} antigen is virtually present on all erythrocytes that are C (rh') positive and/or D (Rh_0) positive.

Most sera that are thought to contain anti-C (rh') and anti-D (Rh_0) actually are composed of anti-D (Rh_0) and anti-G (rh^G) or anti-D (Rh_0), anti-C (rh'), and anti-G (rh^G). These facts have explained the apparent formation of anti-CD in cde/cde (rr) mothers whose husbands and babies are D (Rh_0) positive, C (rh') negative. In reality the antibody is anti-D **(Rh_0)** and anti-G **(rh^G)** rather than anti-D **(Rh_0)** and anti-C **(rh')**.

■ **Discuss the LW antigen.**

LW is a high-incidence antigen that is found on the erythrocytes of humans and monkeys and is not present on the cells of rabbits and guinea pigs. LW stands for Landsteiner and Weiner; they were the first to produce antibodies to this antigen in animals. Antibodies to this antigen are produced in rabbits and guinea pigs when immunized with human or monkey erythrocytes. A few LW-negative individuals with anti-LW have been found. The gene *(LW)* responsible for LW antigen is independent of the genes responsible for Rh antigens. The production of LW and Rh antigens, however, requires common precursor substances. All individuals without detectable Rh antigens, Rh null, have to date been LW negative. LW-negative individuals may have a normal Rh antigen composition or may be Rh null. Giblett has proposed the following genetic pathway.

$$\text{Precursor substance 1} \xrightarrow[\text{blocked by } X^0r/X^0r]{X'r} \text{Precursor substance 2} \xrightarrow[\text{blocked by Rh null/null}]{\text{Rh genes}}$$

$$\text{Rh antigens} \xrightarrow[\text{blocked by } lw/lw]{LW \text{ gene}} \text{LW antigens}$$

Rare individuals who are homozygous for Rh null will have no detectable Rh antigen or LW antigens, whereas individuals homozygous for the *lw* gene *(lwlw)* will lack only the LW antigen and will have a normal complement of Rh antigens.

■ **What is the antigen f (hr) (Rh$_6$)?**

Antigen f (hr) (Rh$_6$) is a compound Rh antigen present on the erythrocytes of individuals who have inherited a chromosome that contains both a *c (hr')* and *e (hr")* gene; e.g., *cDe (R^0)*, *cde (r)*, *cD^{u}e*. This antigen f, sometimes called ce, is detected by anti-f. This antibody is useful in genotyping individuals who have the same phenotype— such as *R^{z}r (CDE/cde)* and *R^{1}R^2 CDe/cDE*. Erythrocytes with the former genotype will react with anti-f (hr) (Rh$_6$), whereas the latter will not.

■ **Describe the antibodies of the Rh blood group system.**

Naturally occurring antibodies. Naturally occuring antibodies of the Rh blood group system have been described only in isolated instances. The most common naturally occurring antibody in the Rh system is anti-rh" (E). These are primarily IgM antibodies reacting with saline-suspended cells. Weak naturally occurring incomplete anti-Rh$_0$ (D) has been recorded. To be classified as a naturally occurring antibody, it must be in a person who has never been a recipient of blood or pregnant.

Immune antibodies. Immune antibodies to all of the Rh factors (antigens) except Hr$_0$ (d) have been described. They are found in certain individuals following a blood transfusion or a pregnancy in which they are exposed to a foreign agglutinogen (antigen). Rh$_0$ (D) is the most potent Rh antigen, followed by hr' (c), rh' (C), rh" (E), and hr" (e).

Rh antibodies are generally IgM saline-reacting when they first appear following immunization. Subsequently, incomplete primarily IgG antibodies develop. They are detectable by the antihuman globulin, enzyme, and high-protein methods. They react best at 37° C. Rh antibodies do not fix complement and therefore are not hemolytic.

■ **Discuss the antihuman globulin test (Coombs' test).**

The antihuman globulin test is used to detect the presence of nonagglutinating antibodies attached to the surface of the RBCs. The antibodies are globulins. The antihuman globulin serum, which is the reagent used in the test, is produced by injecting animals with human globulin.

Nonagglutinating antibodies may attach to RBCs in a variety of clinical situations, such as autoimmune hemolytic anemia, hemolytic disease of the newborn, and hemolytic transfusion reactions, and following certain medications, such as alpha methyldopa, penicillin, cephalothin, and quinidine.

The direct antihuman globulin test detects the in vivo attachment of nonagglutinating antibodies to RBCs. The patient's cells are washed well to remove all traces of plasma proteins and then are reacted with the antihuman globulin serum. Agglutination occurs following centrifugation if the RBCs are coated with nonagglutinating antibodies. The antihuman globulin forms intracellular bridges between the sensitized cells and causes agglutination.

The indirect antihuman globulin test is used to detect the presence of nonagglutinating antibodies present in serum. Serum with suspected antibodies is incubated at 37° C for at least 15 minutes with group O reagent RBCs that contain as many common red blood antigens as possible. Following adequate washing, the RBCs are reacted with the antihuman globulin serum. Agglutination of the RBCs following centrifugation indicates that nonagglutinating RBC antibodies are present in the serum in question.

Antihuman globulin serum can be polyspecific in that it has anti-IgG activity as well as activity against other globulins and some of the components of complement, such as C3 and C4. Most antihuman globulin sera used routinely in blood banks are of this type. Many investigators do not believe that the anticomplement activity is important for routine blood bank work and favor pure anti-IgG antihuman globulin serum.

Monospecific antihuman globulin sera are available to detect IgG, IgA, IgM, C3, and C4. The latter four serums must never be used alone in blood bank work. They are used primarily to identify the specific type of protein coating the RBCs, whether it be IgG, IgA, IgM, C3, or C4. This is most useful in evaluating a positive direct antihuman globulin test.

■ **What is unusual about the Xg blood group system?**

The Xg blood group, described first in 1961, is unusual in that it represents the only known blood group system in which the genes are carried on the X chromosome. The gene Xg^a is responsible for the antigen Xg[a], which is present in about 89% of females and 66% of males. An allele, Xg, has been postulated; however, no antibodies to this proposed antigen have been detected. Anti-**Xg**[a] is detected by the antihuman globulin technique. Females can be of the genotype Xg^aXg^a, Xg^aXg, or $XgXg$, whereas males can be either Xg^a or Xg.

■ **What is the practical importance of the I blood group system?**

The antigens of the I blood group system are I and i. The I antigen is a public antigen, and adults negative for this antigen are extremely rare. Umbilical cord blood, on the other hand, is only weakly reactive to anti-**I**. During the first year and a half of life, erythrocytes become more strongly reactive to anti-**I** and less reactive to anti-**i**.

Anti-**I**, a cold agglutinin, is present in very low titers in the serum of most healthy adults. During and following atypical pneumonia caused by *Mycoplasma pneumoniae,* the cold agglutinin titer may increase manyfold. High titers of anti-**I** are also found in those rare individuals (<0.01%) whose erythrocytes are I negative (ii). Certain autoimmune hemolytic anemias that are present in elderly individuals are caused by the presence of potent auto–anti-**I**. These individuals often have malignancies involving the reticuloendothelial system.

There may be considerable difficulty crossmatching blood for an individual with anti-**I**, because this antibody will react with all red cells including the cells of the patient. It is an IgM that reacts best with saline-suspended erythrocytes at 4° C. Autoabsorption techniques may be required to rid the specimen of this antibody before performing the crossmatches. Autoabsorption, however, should not be done in patients who have recently had transfusions, because the transfused cells may remove alloantibodies. A check for decreased reactivity with cord cells may also be done to help specify the antibody.

■ **Briefly identify and discuss the importance of some of the other blood group systems.**

The human erythrocyte possesses numerous other antigens besides those of the ABO and Rh systems. Two events led to the discovery of the many blood group systems. The first was the widespread utilization of transfusion therapy starting in the early 1940s. The second was the development of the antihuman globulin test in 1945 by Coombs, Mourant, and Race.

1. **MNSs blood group system**– 1927, Landsteiner and Levine
   Importance: Hemolytic disease of the newborn (HDN), transfusion reactions (TR), and paternity
   Incidence: 78% M positive
   72% N positive
2. **P blood group system**– 1927, Landsteiner and Levine
   Importance: TR
   Incidence: 79% P_1 positive
3. **Lutheran blood group system**– 1945, Callendar, Race, and Poykoc
   Importance: HDN, TR
   Incidence: 99.9% Lu^b positive
   8% Lu^a positive
4. **Lewis blood group**– 1946, Mourant
   Importance: TR
   Incidence: 23% Le^a positive
   74% Le^b positive

4% Le^a negative (whites)
23% Le^a and Le^b negative (blacks)

5. **Kell blood group system** — 1946, Coombs, Mourant, and Race
   Importance: HDN, TR
   Incidence: 9% K (Kell) positive
   99.8% k (Cellano) positive
   2% Kp^a (Penny) positive
   99.9% Kp^b (Rautenberg) positive
   0.1% Js^a (Sutter) positive (whites)
   19% Js^a (Sutter) positive (blacks)
   99% Js^b (Sutter) positive

6. **Duffy blood group system** — 1950, Cutbush, Mollison, and Parkin
   Importance: HDN, TR
   Incidence: 66% Fy^a positive (whites)
   10% Fy^a positive (blacks)
   83% Fy^b positive (whites)
   23% Fy^b positive (blacks)
   68% Fy^a and Fy^b negative (blacks)

7. **Kidd blood group system** — 1951, Allen, Diamond, and Niedziela
   Importance: HDN, TR
   Incidence: 77% Jk^a positive
   73% Jk^b positive
   93% Jk^a positive (blacks)

8. **Diego blood group** — 1958, Giblett
   Importance: HDN
   Incidence: 100% Di^a negative (whites)
   36% Di^a positive (South American Indians)
   10% Di^a positive (Chinese and Japanese)

9. **Auberger blood group** — 1961, Salmon, Liberge, Andre, Tippett, and Sanger
   Importance: Potential HDN and TR; only one example of anti-**Au**^{a} has been found
   Incidence: 82% Au positive (whites)

10. **Xg blood group system** — 1962, Mann and associates
    Importance: A sex-linked blood group system with the responsible gene carried on the X chromosome
    Incidence: 89% of females Xg^a positive
    67% of males Xg^a positive

11. **Dombrock system** — 1964, Swanson, Tippett, and Sanger
    Importance: Potential TR
    Incidence: 64% Do^a positive

12. **Colton blood group system** — 1967, Heist and associates
    Importance: Potential TR
    Incidence: 99.7% Co^a positive
    10% Co^b positive

13. **Public antigens** — other red cell antigens with an incidence greater than 99%: Vel, I, Yt^a, Ge, Sm, Chido, Lan, Gy^a, Gn^a, At^a

14. **Private antigens** — antigens found only in members of certain families: Levay, Jobbins, Becker, Van, Wr^a, Be^a, Good, Webb, Swann, Bu, Tr^a, Wb, and others

■ What is the T receptor (antigen)?

All human red cells contain a latent T antigen that can be activated by enzymes produced by certain bacteria. T-activated cells are agglutinated by anti-**T,** present in all human sera except that of the newborn. These cells are not agglutinated by their own serum. T-activation (Hübener-Thomsen-Friedenreich phenomenon) results in polyagglutinable red cells and difficulty in red cell grouping.

■ **What is the HLA complex?**

The HLA complex comprises multiple antigens in various body tissues, including the leukocytes and platelets. Antibodies that react with the antigens of this complex are responsible for febrile transfusion reactions and rejection of homografts. The antigens are determined by genes located on the no. 6 chromosomes. Four distinct subloci have been defined: HLA-A, HLA-B, HLA-C, and HLA-D. The first three loci can be defined by specific HLA antisera and the last by the mixed leukocyte reaction. The present nomenclature was devised by the Histocompatibility Nomenclature Committee of WHO in 1977. Alleles are assigned by specific numbers prefixed by the letters that identify their locus, e.g., HLA-A1. Newly defined or unproven alleles are indicated by an additional prefix (W) inserted between the locus letter and the specified number (HLA-BW22). CW1, CW2, CW3, and CW4 have been defined, but in order to avoid confusion with the complement system symbols, the W will be retained. The HLA alleles are listed in Table 8. HLA-A2 is the most common A allele, and HLA-B12 is the most common B allele.

Table 8. HLA alleles

A locus				
HLA-A1	HLA-A10	HLA-A28	HLA-AW24	HLA-AW33
HLA-A2	HLA-A11	HLA-A29	HLA-AW30	HLA-AW34
HLA-A3	HLA-A25	HLA-AW19	HLA-AW31	HLA-AW36
HLA-A9	HLA-A26	HLA-AW23	HLA-AW32	HLA-AW43

B locus				
HLA-B4	HLA-B14	HLA-BW16	HLA-BW42	HLA-BW50
HLA-B5	HLA-B15	HLA-BW21	HLA-BW44	HLA-BW51
HLA-B6	HLA-B17	HLA-BW22	HLA-BW45	HLA-BW52
HLA-B7	HLA-B18	HLA-BW35	HLA-BW46	HLA-BW53
HLA-B8	HLA-B27	HLA-BW38	HLA-BW47	HLA-BW54
HLA-B12	HLA-B37	HLA-BW39	HLA-BW48	
HLA-B13	HLA-B40	HLA-BW41	HLA-BW49	

C locus		D locus	
HLA-CW1	HLA-CW4	HLA-DW1	HLA-DW4
HLA-CW2	HLA-CW5	HLA-DW2	HLA-DW5
HLA-CW3	HLA-CW6	HLA-DW3	HLA-DW6

■ **Discuss the inheritance of the HLA complex.**

The HLA genes are located on the no. 6 pair of autosomal chromosomes. Each of the chromosomes contains four closely linked HLA subloci. The four genes located on the same chromosome are called a haplotype and, with rare exceptions, segregate together. The two chromosomes segregate independently. The gamete from each parent contributes four of the eight antigens in the child. Since the maternal and paternal haplotypes segregate independently, there is a 1 in 4 probability that children of a mating will have identical HLA types, a 1 in 2 probability that they will share one haplotype, and a 1 in 4 probability that they will not share a haplotype. A child must obtain one haplotype from each of his parents. An example of the inheritance of the HLA-A and HLA-B types is given below. These loci have been studied extensively and can be utilized in paternity exclusion studies.

Children possible

The most frequent haplotypes in whites are HLA-A1, B8; HLA-A2, B12; and HLA-A3, B7.

■ **List some of the criteria for blood donor selection.**
  A. Health: exclude potential donors with chronic disease of heart, lungs, kidneys, or liver or history of cancer
  B. Age: 17 through 65 years
  C. Temperature: must not exceed 99.6° F
  D. Hemoglobin or hematocrit:
     1. Males—exclude those with less than 13.5 gm hemoglobin/dl or less than 41% hematocrit
     2. Females—exclude those with less than 12.5 gm hemoglobin/dl or less than 38% hematocrit
  E. Pulse: must be regular and between 50 and 100 beats per minute

   F. Blood pressure: must be between 90 and 180 mm Hg systolic and 50 and 100 mm Hg diastolic
   G. Pregnancy: exclude those pregnant as well as those pregnant within past 6 weeks
   H. Dental surgery: exclude if less than 72 hours before time of anticipated donation
   I. Recipient of blood or blood component: exclude if received less than 6 months before anticipated donation
   J. Infectious disease:
      1. Viral hepatitis excluded permanently
      2. Malaria—donations must be deferred for 3 years after patients become asymptomatic and after cessation of therapy
      3. Syphilis: exclude if serologic test is positive
   K. Immunization: donations are acceptable:
      1. 24 hours after immunization with toxoids or killed viral, bacterial, or rickettsial vaccines (e.g., tetanus, diphtheria, influenza, and polio [Salk])
      2. 2 weeks after measles, oral polio, mumps, yellow fever, or rabies vaccine
      3. 2 weeks after an immune smallpox reaction or after the scab has fallen off of a primary smallpox reaction
      4. 2 months after German measles vaccine
   L. Weight: must be greater than 110 pounds for full 450 ml donation

■ **Describe the collection of blood from a donor.**

The phlebotomist must be trained and under the supervision of a licensed physician, who must be available for consultation during blood collection. A system of numeric identification must be used so that it will be possible to relate the donor record, the unit of blood, and the pilot tube. Before phlebotomy, the blood container and the pilot tube must be numerically identified and the pilot tube attached to the collection container.

Both arms must be inspected for evidence of recent venipunctures and other lesions. Venipuncture is performed only after adequate preparation of the skin to assure asepsis and a sterile product.

The blood container must be sterile and contain sufficient anticoagulant for the amount of blood to be collected. The unit must be continually mixed during collection and collected within 7 minutes. This is especially important if components are to be prepared. Following collection, the blood must be promptly refrigerated between 1°

and 6° C. Units to be utilized for platelets should not be refrigerated but immediately centrifuged and processed.

Specific instructions for the prevention and treatment of donor reaction must be readily available. Donors must be instructed in possible postphlebotomy reaction such as syncope and should be closely observed for at least 15 minutes before leaving the blood bank.

■ **What procedures are performed on blood that is to be utilized for transfusion purposes?**

The ABO type is determined by (1) testing the red cells with antisera meeting FDA standards and (2) testing the serum for expected antibodies with known A_1 and B red cells. Both results must be in agreement. The Rh_0 (D) type must be determined using anti-Rh_0 (D) serum meeting requirements of the FDA. Tests designed to detect weak $\Re h_0$ variants (D^u) must be performed on all blood initially typed as Rh_0 (D) negative. Routine determination of additional Rh factors need not be done.

All donor sera must be tested for the presence of unexpected antibodies using reagent RBCs meeting FDA standards and using techniques able to demonstrate significant agglutinating, hemolyzing, and coating antibodies. In addition to the above, all blood must be tested for syphilis by an acceptable serologic test and for the hepatitis B antigen. A positive finding in either case is reason for not using the blood for transfusion purposes.

■ **What procedures are performed on recipient blood before transfusion?**

The first and most important step in the preparation of blood for transfusion purposes is to correctly identify the recipient and adequately label the recipient blood sample at the time it is collected. If possible, the potential recipient of blood should be asked to spell his name. This name along with the hospital and room number, date and hour the specimen was obtained, and initials of the phlebotomist must be placed on a label, which must be firmly affixed to the sample tube before leaving the recipient. An error in recipient identification may be fatal.

The ABO and Rh type are determined for the recipient sample using reagents and methods as described for donor, except that testing for $\Re h_0$ variant (D^u) need not be done. Testing with anti-Rh_0 (D) must include an autocontrol (recipient serum-recipient cells) to avoid incorrectly designating an Rh_0 (D)–negative recipient as Rh_0 (D) positive.

The recipient's serum must also be tested for the presence of unexpected antibodies using reagent blood cells that meet FDA requirements. Blood bank records of previous hospital admissions must be readily available so that they may be compared with the results of current testing.

A "major crossmatch" (recipient serum–donor cells) must be performed before transfusion and should include techniques that are able to demonstrate significant hemolyzing, agglutinating, and coating antibodies. The technique must utilize antihuman globulin sera.

A "minor crossmatch" need not be done, since both the recipient and donor sera are tested for regular and irregular antibodies.

■ **What is the so-called type and screen?**

The type and screen procedure determines the patient's ABO and Rh_0 (D) type as well as the presence of unexpected antibodies in the serum. It is a safe substitute for the "routine" one- and two-unit crossmatch that is often ordered for procedures that usually do not require transfusions (e.g., cholecystectomy, thyroidectomy, hysterectomy). If a type and screen procedure has been performed before surgery, fully crossmatched blood can be provided in about 30 minutes. In those rare instances of unexpected, acute, massive blood loss in which the clinical situation does not permit time for a full crossmatch, the type and a negative screen assure that uncrossmatched, type-specific blood can be transfused with safety.

The type and screen will help decrease the incidence of outdating the blood, save money for the patient, and improve the utilization and availability of blood without jeopardizing the patient.

■ **Discuss the proper method of administration of blood and its components.**

The person responsible for the administration of blood obtains a properly labeled unit of blood or blood component from the blood bank. The label attached to the blood must include the recipient's name, hospital and room number, the result of the compatibility tests, the signature of the individual who performed the compatibility tests, and the date performed. A transfusion record must also be provided by the blood bank with each unit to be transfused. This record, a copy of which must be placed on the recipient's chart and a copy sent to the blood bank following completion of the transfusion, must include the following information: recipient's name, hospital or other identification number, results of ABO and Rh testing of both recipient and donor, results of compatibility testing, and signature of person performing them. It should also include space for the signature of the person administering the blood, attesting to the fact that the recipient was properly identified and that the information on the unit label and transfusion record is correct. The record should also provide a space to indicate whether a reaction occurred.

After the proper identification of the recipient and donor blood, the transfusion should be administered through a sterile transfusion set containing a filter to retain coagulated material and other precipitate that could harm the recipient. Under no circumstances should medication be added to blood.

A responsible individual should be in constant attendance for at least the first 15 minutes of each transfusion and at regular intervals thereafter.

The rate of transfusion should be determined by the physician. During the first 15 minutes of observation, the rate should not exceed 5 ml/min. If no adverse reactions are detected, the rate may be increased to 10 ml/min so that the unit is infused in 45 to 90 minutes. If the cardiac status is in question or the patient is severely chronically anemic (Hb of 5 gm or less), the rate should not exceed 1 ml/lb/hr and should be given only as red cells.

■ **Discuss hemolytic disease of the newborn; include its pathogenesis.**

Hemolytic disease of the newborn is a disease in which immune destruction and decreased survival of fetal erythrocytes occur because of interaction of these erythrocytes with maternal IgG isoagglutinins that have crossed the placenta. The infant may exhibit anemia, edema, hepatosplenomegaly, hyperbilirubinemia, and, in severe cases, central nervous system damage (kernicterus) and even death from heart failure.

Isoimmunization of mothers may occur following transplacental passage of fetal erythrocytes into the maternal circulation during the last trimester of pregnancy and at the time of separation of the placenta following delivery. Sensitization may also follow blood transfusion.

Hemolytic disease of the newborn can result from fetomaternal incompatibilities in the Rh, ABO, Kell, Duffy, and other blood group systems. The first two are the most common, and Rh_0 (D) hemolytic disease is generally the severest. ABO hemolytic disease of the newborn occurs almost exclusively in group A or B infants born to group O mothers, whereas Rh hemolytic disease occurs most commonly in Rh_0 (D)−positive infants born to sensitized Rh_0 (D)−negative mothers.

■ **Describe prenatal evaluation for hemolytic disease of the newborn.**

There are three avenues available for the correct prenatal assessment of the severity of possible hemolytic disease of the newborn: (1) history of the fate of previous infants, (2) erythrocyte antigen and serum and antibody studies, and (3) amniotic fluid studies. No one avenue is adequate, and all three may be necessary to correctly evaluate the individual situation. The following laboratory studies are suggested for proper evaluation of this problem.

A. At 6 weeks' gestational age or first prenatal visit
   1. Obtain ABO and Rh type to include D^u of all mothers.
   2. Screen mother's serum for irregular isoagglutinins using reagent red cells.
   3. Identify irregular isoagglutinins, if any are detected, using panel of reagent red cells.
   4. If mother is Rh_0 (D) negative, determine father's ABO type and probable Rh genotype.
   5. Freeze and save mother's serum for future retiter or reference.

B. At 24 to 28 weeks' gestation
   1. Rescreen mother's serum for irregular isoagglutinins.
   2. If irregular isoagglutinins are present, identify and titer in parallel with previous serum samples.

C. At 22 and 32 weeks' gestational age in women with demonstrable antibodies
   1. Perform amniocentesis for spectrophotometric analysis of amniotic fluid (a) for baseline studies and (b) to detect severely involved infants for whom delivery at 32 to 37 weeks or intrauterine transfusion could offer a chance for survival.
   2. Determine ABO type of the amniotic fluid of secretor infants by hemagglutination inhibition.
   3. Identify red cells recovered from amniotic fluid by ABO type, Rh type, and direct antihuman globulin test.

D. At 24 to 36 weeks' gestational age
   1. Repeat amniocentesis at 2-week intervals to evaluate need for intrauterine transfusion or premature delivery.

E. At 34 to 35 weeks' gestational age
   1. Rescreen mother's serum for irregular isoagglutinins; especially important in Rh_0 (D)–negative mothers.

F. Before delivery of mother with irregular isoagglutinins
   1. The blood bank should be notified of impending delivery as

soon as possible so that blood may be immediately available at delivery for exchange tranfusion if indicated.

■ **Discuss prevention of maternal Rh_0 (D) sensitization.**

Levine recognized that Rh_0 (D) sensitization is more common in ABO-compatible matings than in incompatible matings. Subsequent observations and studies revealed that Rh_0 (D) sensitization is prevented if IgG anti-**Rh_0 (D)** is administered to the mother within 72 hours of delivery of a Rh_0 (D)–positive child or following miscarriage or therapeutic abortion. This passive immunization is 98% to 99.5% effective in preventing sensitization to Rh_0 (D).

The following should be performed for maximum benefit from anti-**Rh_0(D)** immunoglobulin therapy.

1. Determine Rh_0 (D) type (including D^u) on all expectant mothers.
2. Screen all Rh_0 (D)–negative mothers for irregular isoagglutinins.
3. Determine Rh_0 (D) type (including D^u) on cord blood from babies of Rh_0 (D)–negative mothers.
4. Perform direct antihuman globulin test on cord blood.

The mother is a candidate for the anti-**Rh_0 (D)** immunoglobulin therapy if the following criteria are met: (a) she is Rh_0 (D) negative and D^u negative; (b) she is not immunized to the Rh_0 (D) factor, as determined after delivery; (c) the baby is Rh_0 (D) positive or D^u positive; and (d) the baby has a negative direct antihuman globulin test. The mother is still a candidate if the baby has a positive direct antihuman globulin test because of an antibody other than anti-**Rh_0(D)**.

A dose of 1 ml ($300\mu g$) of anti-**Rh_0 (D)** immunoglobulin is given intramuscularly to the mother following a compatible minor crossmatch. An incompatible crossmatch and/or positive maternal D^u in a mother previously determined to be Rh_0 (D) and D^u negative may indicate a massive transplacental hemorrhage, necessitating more than a 1-ml dose. The magnitude of the fetal-maternal hemorrhage may be estimated with the Kleihauer acid elution test by identifying fetal red cells in the maternal blood. Fetal cells contain fetal hemoglobin, which resists acid elution.

Therapy should also be given to Rh_0 (D)–negative women following miscarriage or therapeutic abortion. A 50-μg dose of anti-**Rh_0 (D)** immunoglobulin has been found effective for first-trimester abortions.

■ **Discuss anmiocentesis as a tool in monitoring suspected hemolytic disease of the newborn.**

In 1953 Bevis first suggested that examination of amniotic fluid could give valuable information in the evaluation of an unborn child with potential hemolytic disease of the newborn. This concept was further expanded by Liley and others in the early 1960s. After the amniotic fluid is obtained, it must be protected from light and clarified by centifugation. The fluid is then scanned in a narrow-band spectrophotometer to determine the presence of a 450-nm absorption peak, which represents breakdown products of hemoglobin. A normal amniotic fluid scan has no significant 450-nm peak, whereas fluid from a pregnancy with hemolytic disease has an absorption peak with a 450-nm maximum.

The severity of the hemolytic disease can be assessed by the net density of the 450-nm peak. Liley plotted optical density versus gestational age and developed three zones of involvment. Zone 1 peaks indicate mild or no involvement; zone 2 peaks suggest moderate involvement requiring careful observation and follow up; zone 3 peaks suggest severe disease, usually requiring intrauterine transfusions or immediate delivery of the child. Amniotic fluid studies are also utilized to determine fetal maturity, sex, fetal blood groups, and chromosomal and biochemical abnormalities.

■ **Discuss selection of blood for a newborn with hemolytic disease of the newborn.**

Blood selected for transfusion therapy of the newborn must be compatible with serum from the mother. Subsequent tranfusions must be compatible with serum of both the mother and the baby. Antibodies present in the newborn's serum are present in the maternal serum in invariably greater quantities. Utilization of maternal serum also enables the blood bank to obtain and crossmatch blood for the baby before delivery.

It is preferable to use blood that is less than 3 but no more than 5 days old. An attempt should be made to use, if possible, blood that is of the same ABO group as the baby and that is negative for the offending antigen. When the mother is group O, group O blood must be used. In the latter situation, if the child is other than group O, red cells or hemolysin-free whole blood should be given.

■ **What are the indications for transfusion therapy?**

Blood and blood component therapy can be lifesaving and at other times a valuable therapeutic procedure. However, because of hidden dangers that may be present, a prescription for blood or component therapy should be made only with justifiable indication. Component rather than whole blood therapy should be utilized so that more than one patient may be treated with a single donation. Following are the major indications:

1. To maintain blood volume and treat hypovolemic shock. Severe, massive, acute blood loss is probably the only indication for whole blood therapy.
2. To improve oxygen-carrying capacity. This is best treated with RBCs rather than whole blood.
3. To replace platelets and other coagulation factors that are deficient in persons with hemorrhagic disorders.
4. Exchange transfusion to treat newborns with hemolytic disease and persons with hepatic coma.

■ **Discuss RBCs.**

RBCs are prepared from whole blood by removing two thirds of the plasma-anticoagulant solution so that the hematocrit is about 60% to 70%. This separation is accomplished by sedimentation or centrifugation. If separation is done in a closed system, the RBCs may be transfused up to 21 days from the date of collection.

RBCs should be utilized whenever the indication is to improve oxygen-carrying capacity. In addition to being an efficient method of achieving this, RBCs reduce the possibility of circulatory overload. They also contain less sodium, acid, potassium, and ammonia than whole blood and are less likely to aggravate cardiac, renal, and hepatic failures when they exist.

■ **Discuss the use of platelet concentrates.**

Platelet concentrates are administered to individuals who are bleeding as a result of thrombocytopenia. The platelet count is usually less than 20,000/cu mm. A patient with a low platelet count and no evidence of bleeding probably should not be treated. Individuals who require surgery should have at least 50,000 platelets per cubic millimeter.

Platelets are obtained by differential centrifugation of whole blood or by plateletpheresis of a single donor. The platelet yield of the former technique is about 0.6×10^{11} platelets per unit and about 5 to 7 $\times 10^{11}$ by the latter method. The expiration time of platelets is 72 hours after collection.

Whenever possible, platelets from ABO- and Rh_0 (D)–compatible donors should be used. In the event that platelets from Rh_0 (D)–positive donors must be transfused into an Rh_0 (D)–negative recipient, the recipient should also be given anti-**Rh_0 (D)** immunoglobulin to prevent Rh_0 (D) sensitization due to the Rh_0 (D)–positive RBCs present in the platelet concentrate.

The usual dose is 4 to 12 units of platelets, depending on the platelet count and the size of the patient. A unit of platelets will usually increase the platelet count by 7,000 to 10,000/cu mm/sq m of body surface area.

The patient's response to platelet transfusion should be monitored with posttransfusion platelet counts at 1 and 24 hours. If a patient is refractory to platelets from random donors, the use of HLA-compatible platelets should be considered if they are available.

■ **Discuss cryoprecipitate.**

Cryoprecipitate contains primarily factor VIII and some fibrinogen. It is prepared by thawing fresh-frozen plasma between 2° and 6° C. After centrifugation, the supernatant plasma is removed and the cryoprecipitate that remains is refrozen. When needed for transfusion, it is thawed at 37° C and dissolved in 10 ml of saline solution. Each unit of cryoprecipitate contains about 80 to 120 units of factor VIII. A unit of factor VIII is defined as the factor VIII activity in 1 ml of fresh normal plasma.

Cryoprecipitate is used in the treatment of hemorrhage occurring in hemophilia. It has also been used in the treatment of hypofibrinogenemia. Superconcentrates of factor VIII containing up to 1,000 units per container are available commercially.

■ **Discuss frozen RBCs.**

The shelf life of RBCs can be extended almost indefinitely by freezing and storing at ultralow temperatures in the presence of a cryoprotective agent such as glycerol. At the time of use, the cells must be thawed and washed to remove the glycerol and transfused within 24 hours. Presently, because of cost, the use of frozen RBCs is limited, but as technology advances, freezing will probably become the prime method of storage. Massachusetts General Hospital, Boston, and Cook County Hospital, Chicago, are now almost exclusively using frozen red cells.

■ **What are some of the hazards of transfusion therapy?**

Adverse reactions can be divided into immediate and delayed types. A reaction is any unfavorable symptom experienced by the recipient. An immediate reaction occurs within minutes or hours after start of a transfusion, whereas a delayed reaction occurs days or weeks after a transfusion.

A. Immediate reactions
1. Hemolytic transfusion reactions
   a. Hemolysis related to blood group incompatibility
   b. Hemolysis related to faulty administration of blood through 5% dextrose solution or 5% dextrose in 0.25% saline solution
2. Reactions secondary to administration of bacterially contaminated blood
3. Circulatory overload reactions
4. Pyrogenic reactions
   a. Exogenous pyrogens—bacterial
   b. Endogenous pyrogens—caused by disease state of recipient
   c. Leukoagglutinins—common in females who have had multiple pregnancies
   d. Platelet agglutinins
5. Allergic reactions—hives, bronchospasm, and/or generalized anaphylaxis may occur following administration of blood or plasma containing a protein component to which the recipient is sensitive; serious anaphylactic transfusion reactions occur in individuals with IgA deficiency who have been immunized to IgA
6. Hemorrhagic diathesis following massive transfusions
7. Air embolism—rare since widespread usage of plastic bags
8. Citrate toxicity—(rare) may result in hypocalcemia in individuals with impaired liver function
B. Delayed reactions
1. Transmission of disease
   a. Viral hepatitis
   b. Syphilis
   c. Malaria
   d. Chagas' disease
   e. Brucellosis
2. Isosensitization—may prevent or make difficult transfusion therapy in the future, as well as placing in jeopardy the fate of future children of women of childbearing age
3. Transfusional siderosis—follows transfusion of large quantities of blood over prolonged periods (Remember: each unit of blood contains 250 mg of iron.)

■ **Why is CPD anticoagulation and preservation of blood superior to that of ACD?**

Until recently, blood obtained for transfusion purposes was drawn almost exclusively into acid-citrate-dextrose (ACD) solution. This solution is an anticoagulant and preservative allowing a shelf life of 21 days, which is the maximum storage time that 70% of the red cells will survive 24 hours in a recipient when transfused.

The oxygen dissociation curve of blood preserved in ACD solution shifts significantly to the left ($\downarrow P_{50}$). Therefore, ACD blood has a decreased ability to release oxygen to the tissues, because the affinity of hemoglobin for oxygen is increased.

The concentration of the red cell 2,3-diphosphoglycerate (2,3-DPG) is inversely proportional to the affinity of hemoglobin for oxygen. During storage of blood in ACD, the concentration of red cell, 2,3-DPG decreases and the affinity of hemoglobin for oxygen is increased.

Studies of blood drawn into citrate-phosphate-dextrose (CPD) solution have shown that the 24-hour 70% red cell survival is maintained for 28 days following collection. More important, blood collected in CPD retains a higher 2,3,-DPG concentration for a longer period of time, resulting in a lesser shift to the left in the oxygen dissociation curve. Thus, hemoglobin will more readily release oxygen to the tissues.

The above are a few reasons why the anticoagulant-preservative of choice is CPD. Major blood banks throughout the country have changed to this anticoagulant. The FDA has licensed CPD blood for only a 21-day "out date," similar to that for ACD blood. Rejuvenating solutions containing substances such as pyruvate, inosine, adenine, and phosphate may in the future be utilized to improve the 24-hour posttransfusion survival of red cells.

The viability of red cells following transfusions is dependent on their adenosine triphosphate (ATP) level. If added to CPD, adenine, an aminopurine, will prolong and maintain the level of ATP so that the blood can be used for up to 35 days after collection. CPD-adenine has recently been approved by the FDA for collection of blood for human use in the United States. Its use has not yet been approved for preparing platelets.

CHAPTER 4

Urinology

Opal Kelly

■ **Why do we measure pH of urine?**

pH is a measurement of free hydrogen (H^+) ions in the urine. It reflects the ability of the kidney to maintain normal H^+ ion concentration in the plasma and extracellular fluid (ECF). Urine pH will range from 4.5 to 8.0. Knowledge of pH in a fresh urine specimen may be of assistance in evaluating metabolic disorders. Urine is very acid in diabetic ketoacidosis. In renal tubular acidosis (RTA) the urine is persistently neutral to alkaline. In potassium deficiency the pH tends to rise. In some urinary tract infections, in which a "urea splitting" organism is present, an alkaline urine is formed.

■ **What are the ketone bodies?**

When there is a defect in carbohydrate metabolism or inadequate carbohydrate in the diet, the body produces increasing amounts of fatty acids for the bulk of its energy needs and generates an excess of acetylcoenzyme A that cannot be oxidized to water and Co_2 or be disposed of in other metabolic routes. This results in the increased formation of ketone bodies, which are excreted in the urine. The three ketone bodies present in urine are beta-hydroxybutyric acid (78%), acetoacetic acid (20%), and acetone (2%). Acetone is formed by the nonreversible decarboxylation of diacetic acid.

Current test methods detect acetoacetic acid and acetone by their reaction with nitroprusside in the presence of glycine and a buffer. A purple color of varying intensity forms, depending on ketone concentration. The test is more sensitive to acetoacetic acid (diacetic acid) than it is to acetone. Hart's test for the detection of beta-hydroxybutyric acid is rarely used.

Ketonuria occurs most frequently in uncontrolled diabetes mellitus. It may also be seen in acute febrile and toxic states, with vomiting, after anesthesia, and with diets low in carbohydrate.

■ **Why is a test for sugar done?**

Routine testing for sugar may be done using a dipstick, testing only for glucose. The urine should be at room temperature. Using an alkaline copper sulfate, one may test for all reducing substances. Sugars that reduce copper sulfate to cuprous oxide are glucose, lactose, galactose, fructose, and pentose. These sugars may be identified by thin-layer chromatography.

Glucose in the urine with a high blood sugar indicates diabetes mellitus. Glucose in the urine with a normal blood sugar indicates renal glycosuria.

■ **When is occult blood found?**

The occult blood test may be positive when either large numbers of RBCs (hematuria) or hemoglobin (hemoglobinuria) is present. Hemoglobinuria may be caused by intravascular hemolysis, transfusion reaction, or lysis of cells from standing in very dilute urine. Methods used to detect blood are based on the peroxidase activity of hemoglobin. Since myoglobin also has peroxidase activity, it will give a positive reaction for blood if present.

■ **What is the normal excretion of protein per 24 hours?**

Normal urine contains only a small amount of protein, usually less than 100 mg/day. An occasional normal subject will excrete 150 mg/day.

■ **When may proteinuria occur?**

Proteinuria may occur as the result of any of the following: (1) disruption of normal glomerular capillary permeability such as occurs through antigen-antibody complement deposition, as in acute poststreptococcal glomerulonephritis or systemic lupus erythematosus (SLE) with renal involvement; (2) tubular proteinuria—there is an increased excretion of plasma proteins in the presence of a normal glomerulus; the small molecular size of the Bence Jones protein allows it to be readily filtered and excreted in the urine; or (3) the irritative effect of infection, which may result in increased exudation of plasma proteins into the urine; however, this amounts to only a few hundred milligrams per day.

■ **What are some substances that might cause a false-positive reaction when acids are used for qualitative protein determinations?**

Some substances that cause a false-positive protein reaction with the use of acids are x-ray contrast media, tolbutamide, and massive doses of penicillin.

■ **What is orthostatic proteinuria?**

It is an abnormal protein excretion that occurs only in the upright position. There may be as much as 1,000 mg/24 hr. When the individual is at rest, the abnormal protein completely disappears. The precise mechanism is unknown but is considered to be a nonglomerular type of proteinuria and thus not pathologic.

■ **Bence Jones protein in the urine has what unusual characteristic?**

Bence Jones protein, a light-chain protein with a molecular weight of 20,000, is excreted in the urine of patients with multiple myeloma. The protein precipitates at temperatures between 40° and 60° C and redissolves near 100° C. Another test depends on the precipitation of the protein in the cold with salts and acid. Electrophoresis or immunodiffussion are more commonly used today. Bence Jones protein will not be detected by the protein test area on the dipstick. Tests using heat or acid will detect the protein.

■ **When cloudy urines are received, how can they be cleared?**

When urine stands and cools below body temperature, crystals may precipitate and should be dissolved before centrifuging. In acid urine, urates precipitate causing a pink cloud, "brick dust," and can be dissolved by warming the urine to 60° C. In alkaline urine, phosphates form a white cloud and can be dissolved by the addition of a few drops of 5% acetic acid. This will not destroy cells or casts. Cells and casts will be obscured by the amorphous material.

■ **What is the difference between specific gravity and osmolality?**

Specific gravity compares the weight of a liquid with the weight of distilled H_2O and measures the relative amount of solids in the urine. There are technical limitations in using the urinometer to measure specific gravity. Most laboratories now use the refractometer, which measures the angle of refraction of light passing through the urine. This angle is directly proportional to the amount of solids present. This instrument uses little specimen and is temperature compensated. Both instruments are standardized against distilled water. Protein and glucose raise specific gravity. In diabetics the glucose correction may be necessary when doing a concentration test.

Osmolality is the measurement of osmotically active particles. The freezing depression point (FDP) is measured and converted to osmotic pressure. The FDP is the temperature at which a solute changes from a liquid to a solid state. One milliosmol will lower the freezing point −0.00186° C.

■ **What are concentration and dilution?**

They describe the degree to which the nephron changes the solute density above or below that of the plasma ultrafiltrate before it is excreted as urine.

■ **After 12 hours of fluid restriction, what concentration does normal urine reach?**

After fluids have been restricted for 12 to 16 hours, usually over the night hours, the urine should reach a specific gravity of at least 1.025 and an osmolality greater than 800 mOsm.

■ **Why is the microscopic examination of the urine essential?**

The microscopic examination may be called "a liquid biopsy of the kidney." There may be a direct disease relationship to the findings in the urine sediment.

■ **What are casts?**

Casts are molds of the tubule and occur because of "gelling" of the protein. The protein is Tamm-Horsfal, which is apparently secreted by the cells lining the distal part of the nephron. It is readily precipitated in a urine of low pH and high specific gravity. Casts may be absent in chronic renal disease even though proteinuria is significant, because the capacity to form acid and concentrated urine has been lost.

■ **Can the width of a cast be an indication of the severity of renal disease?**

Casts are thought to form in the distal or collecting tubule. Broad casts are probably formed in the collecting tubules. Large numbers of broad casts indicate widespread stasis in the nephron.

■ **How is the width of a cast judged?**

A narrow cast is 1 to 2 RBCs in width; a medium cast is 3 to 4 RBCs in width; and a broad cast is greater than 5 RBCs in width.

■ **What are hyaline casts?**

Hyaline casts are precipitated protein without formed elements. In small numbers they are not clinically significant, but they are associated with proteinuria and therefore are seen in almost every clinical situation.

■ **What are cell casts?**

Epithelial cell casts are composed largely of desquamated epithelial cells as a result of intrinsic renal disease. These casts may be difficult to distinguish from WBC casts unless the structure is intact. Large

numbers of renal epithelial cells and casts containing these cells indicate an active degenerative process involving the tubules. They may
be found in glomerulonephritis, acute tubular necrosis, and active
pyelonephritis.

In WBC casts, the cells have become enmeshed in the protein matrix. They may be found in acute pyelonephritis or noninflammatory
diseases such as acute glomerulonephritis and SLE. The casts should
be carefully distinguished from clumped WBCs.

In RBC casts, the RBCs have become enmeshed in the protein matrix. The cast is usually red-orange. The individual cells may be difficult to identify because they are so tightly packed. The RBC cast is
indicative of glomerulitis.

■ **What are granular casts?**

Granular casts are probably the result of casts "lying in the tubule"
and have degenerated from epithelial cells, WBC or RBC casts, and
protein. Some cellular material may still be evident. They may be
classed as coarse or fine. This does not account for the showers of apparently fresh-formed granular casts that occur abruptly in normal subjects. These casts may also be the result of irregular flocculation of protein.

■ **What are fatty casts?**

Casts containing fat droplets are called "fatty casts." They are found
with oval fat bodies (OFB), free-fat droplets, and heavy proteinuria
and are associated with the nephrotic syndrome.

■ **What is the nephrotic syndrome?**

The nephrotic syndrome is characterized by edema, proteinuria 3 to
4+ qualitatively and greater than 3.5 gm quantitatively, hypoal-
buminemia, and hyperlipemia. Microscopic examination may reveal
the fatty cast, OFB, free-fat droplets, and hyaline and granular casts.
RBCs and tubular epithelial cells are variable. RBC casts are rarely
found. Depending on the cause, renal function may not be markedly
impaired.

Some of the diseases in which the nephrotic syndrome may occur
are glomerulonephritis, diabetic glomerulosclerosis, systemic lupus
erythematosus, and occasionally as the result of allergins, insect bites,
and drugs.

■ **What are some diseases in which RBCs, RBC casts, and protein occur?**

When RBC casts and heavy protein are found, the disease is usually
glomerular: (1) acute poststreptococcal glomerulonephritis; (2) glo-

merulitis associated with disease such as SLE, Goodpasture's syndrome, Schönlein-Henoch purpura, and thrombotic thrombocytopenic purpura; or (3) malignant nephrosclerosis. RBCs and RBC casts without heavy proteinuria may also be found in glomerulonephritis, subacute bacterial endocarditis (SBE), and hereditary nephritis.

■ **When would you find RBCs with minimal proteinuria?**
Proteinuria is minimal with RBCs when there is a focal urinary tract disease: (1) tumor, (2) infection, (3) stone, (4) trauma, (5) polycystic kidney disease, (6) clotting disorders, and (7) sickle cell trait.

■ **What is glomerular filtrate?**
The glomerular filtrate is essentially protein-free and free of all cells. It is composed of water and dissolved solids such as electrolytes, amino acids, urea, and all substances unbound to protein and capable of being in solution.

■ **What properties must a substance have to be suitable for use in measurement of the glomerular filtration rate (GFR)?**
To adequately measure GFR, a substance must be freely filtered and remain fairly constant in transit through the nephron, being neither secreted, reabsorbed, nor diffused.

The substance that best fulfills these requirements is inulin, a fructose polysaccharide. Inulin must be infused at a constant rate during the test. Blood and urine must be collected at precise times. Because of the constant infusion and precise timing of the specimens, its major use is in areas where precision is required. This is called an exogenous clearance.

Endogenous clearance tests measure a substance that occurs naturally in plasma and is excreted in the urine. Creatinine is the substance measured in clinical practice. Endogenous creatinine clearance measured at the same time as inulin appears to accurately reflect GFR at normal and moderately decreased clearances. At very low levels of GFR, creatinine clearance appears to be significantly higher than the GFR.

■ **What is clearance?**
Clearance is the volume of blood plasma completely cleared of a substance in 1 minute by renal excretion.

$$C = \frac{UV}{P}$$

C = Clearance of a substance
U = Urine concentration of a substance
V = Volume of urine collected over a given period of time
P = Mean plasma concentration of a substance during the time of urine formation

■ **What are some of the things necessary for an accurate renal clearance?**

To assure accuracy of renal clearance, the total urine must be collected during a precise period of time. If short clearance periods are used, such as 1 or 2 hours, a brisk urine flow should be established to ensure spontaneous voiding and complete emptying of the bladder. This can be achieved with adequate hydration. If fluids must be restricted because of impaired renal function, longer clearance periods should be used.

■ **What is creatinine clearance (C_{cr})? Why is it preferred?**

Creatinine is a by-product of protein metabolism; it is produced at a constant rate, is freely filtered by the glomerulus, and is considered to be neither secreted nor reabsorbed. Urine should be collected over long periods of time. Twenty-four hours is the best period of time to minimize collection error. Normal C_{cr} is 90 to 140 ml/min/1.73 sq m or 100 to 180 liter/24 hr/1.73 sq m.

Because creatinine is related to muscle mass, it is important to express creatinine excretion in terms of body size. Females excrete 14 to 22 mg/kg/day, and males 20 to 26 mg/kg/day. Serum creatinine is also an index of renal function. The use of serum creatinine in place of creatinine clearance eliminates the error of inaccurate urine collection. Serum creatinine is 0.6 to 1.2 mg/dl in females and 0.8 to 1.4 mg/dl in males.

Creatinine clearance has replaced urea clearance. Urea is partially reabsorbed from the glomerular filtrate. Factors other than GFR affect urea. Low urine flow results in increased urea reabsorption. The optimum urine flow should be greater than 2 ml/min. The daily production of urea is variable and depends partially on protein intake. BUN level rises with accelerated protein breakdown, trauma, infection, steroid therapy, gastrointestinal bleeding, or ingestion of a high protein diet and falls when a person is on a low-protein diet.

■ **When will bilirubin be found?**

Bilirubin is the breakdown product of hemoglobin. It is found in the urine of patients with obstructive jaundice or liver damage caused by exposure to toxins or ingestion of certain drugs. It may appear in the urine of patients with hepatitis before clinical jaundice appears.

■ **When will urobilinogen appear in the urine?**

Urobilinogen is the product of bilirubin oxidation and will be increased in the urine when there is hemolysis of RBCs. It may be increased in liver disease, because the liver cells are not able to reabsorb or reexcrete circulating urobilinogen. It may be absent in the urine when there is complete obstruction of the bile duct. The qualitative test must be performed on fresh urine.

■ **Identify some of the colors of urine.**

Straw, pale, almost watery-appearing urine usually indicates a low specific gravity. Yellow is the normal color of urine and indicates a specific gravity of 1.012 to 1.019 with an output of 1 to 1.5 liters/day. Amber indicates a concentrated urine, with the volume usually under 1 liter/day. Some of the abnormal pigments are brownish yellow or brownish green, which indicates bilirubin; red to red-brown, hemoglobinuria; red-brown with brown pigmented casts in the sediment, myoglobin; and dark brown, methemoglobin. Some foods and drugs will also pigment the urine.

■ **What is an Addis count?**

An Addis count is a quantitative enumeration of RBCs, WBCs, and casts from a urine sample collected over an accurately timed period. A precise amount of urine is centrifuged for an exact length of time and then counted on a counting chamber. It is usually collected overnight after restriction of fluids the day of the test. The accepted length of time is 12 hours but may be shortened to 6 to 9 hours. The urine should be preserved with formalin. The pH should be low and the concentration high.

■ **What are kidney stones?**

Kidney stones are composed of a mucoprotein matrix and inorganic and organic crystals. The most common stone is the calcium oxalate stone, which usually occurs in a sterile urine. There is a familial, probably a genetic, predisposition to form calcium oxalate stones. They may also result from hyperparathyroidism, renal tubular acidosis, and idiopathic hypercalciuria. Other types of stones are uric acid, sometimes found in patients with gout and sometimes caused by increased excretion of urates. Magnesium ammonium phosphate stones reflect chronic urinary tract infection with "urea splitting" organisms.

Cystine stones are always associated with patients who have a genetic defect in tubular transport and reabsorption of dibasic amino acids, cystine, lysine, arginine, and ornithine. Stone formation is probably the result of reduced urine volume and increased excretion of calcium, oxalate, uric acid, or ammonia (phosphate) or of changes conducive to stone formation at normal concentration of crystalloids, pH particularly. At the time stones are being passed there may be small amounts of protein and hematuria, gross to microscopic. With magnesium ammonium phosphate stones, the urine is the same as that in urinary tract infection.

■ **What is the average daily volume of urine in the normal adult?**

The normal daily urine output is from 1 to 1.5 liters. The total output depends on fluid intake.

■ **What is the total amount of solids carried off in the urine daily?**

The total amount of solids ranges from 50 to 70 gm/day, decreasing with age. A large portion of the solute is composed of urea and NaCl, directly related to dietary intake.

■ **What is polyuria?**

Polyuria is a markedly increased excretion of urine, 3 to 4 liters/day. It may be due to increased fluid intake or diuretic medication. Polyuria is found in disease states such as diabetes mellitus and diabetes insipidus. It is a symptom of early chronic renal disease and certain tumors of the brain and spinal cord.

■ **What are oliguria and anuria?**

Oliguria is decreased urine output, less than 400 ml/day. It may be the result of decreased intravascular volume due to hemorrhage (external or concealed), ECF losses, protracted vomiting or diarrhea, burns, or severe congestive heart failure. Oliguria may also be the result of intrinsic renal disease: (1) vascular: renal cortical necrosis; (2) glomerular: acute glomerulonephritis, serum sickness, SLE; (3) interstitial disease: papillary necrosis; (4) tubular disease: acute tubular necrosis as a result of prolonged ischemia due to (a) prerenal azotemia, which may occur during extensive trauma, hemorrhage, surgical procedures, obstetric complications (placenta previa, abruption), and septicemia or (b) nephrotoxins: heavy metals (Hg, Bi, Pb, etc.), anesthetic gases (methoxyflurane [Penthrane]), antibiotics (gentamycin, kanamycin, etc.), myoglobin (muscle injury), hemoglobin (intravascular hemolysis).

Anuria is urinary output of less than 100 ml/day. There may be total cessation of urine due to obstructive uropathy such as stones, prostatism, tumor, or sloughed papillae.

CHAPTER 5

Radiochemistry

Raymond Zastrow

■ **What is a radionuclide?**

A nuclide is any atomic nucleus and its orbital electrons. A radionuclide is a nuclide that emits radioactivity as it forms another nuclide.

■ **What is an isotope?**

An isotope is one or more stable or unstable forms of the same element having the same atomic number. They have the same chemical properties but vary as to radioactive properties.

■ **What types of radiation are useful in radiochemistry?**

There are two basic types of radiation—particle emission and electromagnetic emission.

■ **Explain particle emission.**

During atomic rearrangement (disintegration), depending on the element involved, a variety of atomic subparticles may be emitted. These include electrons from the atomic orbital rings or nuclear derivatives such as alpha particles, beta particles, and positrons.

■ **What is an alpha particle?**

It is a helium nucleus stripped of its orbital ring of electrons. Since it consists of two protons and two neutrons, it has a positive charge and a mass of 4. Because of this heavy mass, as compared with electrons, beta particles, and positrons, its speed is slow, penetration of tissues is short (measured in micra), and it thus remains in contact with local tissue molecules for a comparatively long time. This contact combined with the 2+ charge of the double protons leads to a high probability of interaction with tissue molecules, resulting in their rearrangement. This rearrangement is called ionization.

■ **What are electrons?**

Electrons are high-speed, negatively charged particles arranged in orbital rings about a nucleus. Their weight is $1/1,840$ that of a neutron. Because of the low weight and high speed, the chance for contact with individual tissue items is lessened and the specific ionization is a fraction of that of the alpha particles. The tissue penetration, however, is deeper (measured in millimeters).

■ **What is a beta particle, or negatron?**

Beta particles are negatively charged particles arising from the nucleus secondary to nuclear rearrangement. Their charge, weight, speed, penetration, and specific ionization are identical to those of the electron.

■ **What is a positron?**

Positrons are also nuclear derivatives emitted during disintegration. They carry a positive charge but in all other respects are similar to beta particles.

■ **What are the types of electromagnetic radiation?**

The electromagnetic spectrum includes visible light, radiowaves, microwaves, and so on. The highest frequency electromagnetic spectra are of interest to radiochemistry—the gamma photons and x-ray photons.

■ **What are gamma photons?**

Gamma photons are high-energy, high-frequency electromagnetic forces derived during nuclear rearrangement. They travel at the speed of light and thus have high penetration and low specific ionization.

■ **How do x-rays differ from gamma photons?**

X-rays are derived during orbital electron rearrangements. They also travel at the speed of light and in other respects are similar to gamma photons.

■ **What does the M in technetium-99M mean?**

The suffix M indicates a metastable state. It indicates an atom undergoing decay yet retaining its energy. Technetium (Tc) is a daughter nuclide of molybdenum-99. Its intermediate state is Tc-99M which has a 6-hour half-life.

■ **What is physical half-life ($T^{1/2}$)?**

It is the time required for a radionuclide to decay to one-half the number of original atoms. For example, 1 millicurie of a radionuclide will decay to half a millicurie (500 microcuries) in one half-life.

■ **What is a curie?**

It is a unit of activity defined as 3.7×10^{10} disintegrations per second.

- **What is a millicurie?**
  A millicurie is 10^{-3} curies.
- **What is a microcurie?**
  A microcurie is 10^{-6} curies.
- **What is effective half-life?**
  It is the physical half-life combined with the rate of biologic degradation or biologic half-life.
- **What is specific activity?**
  It is the concentration of radioactive material and is usually expressed as millicuries per gram.
- **What is shielding?**
  Various materials may be used to block the energy photons so that they do not strike the technologist or adjacent instrumentation. The thickness required to reduce the amount of radiation on the side opposite the shield is dependent on the density of the material used.
- **What is the half-value layer?**
  It is the thickness of any given shielding material that will reduce by half the radioactivity on the opposite side from the source.
- **What is a collimator?**
  It is a perforated shield used to protect the detector instrument head from extraneous energy photons while acting to direct the specific detection of a given photon source.
- **What is the inverse square law?**
  Radiation exposure and detection levels decrease with the square of the distance from the source. If the distance between the source and the detector head is doubled, the amount of radiation detected is reduced to one fourth that of the original.
- **What are the cardinal principles of radiation safety?**
  Shielding, distance, physical half-life, good housekeeping, and responsible record-keeping. Housekeeping includes correct waste disposal and placarding of radioactive areas. Good record-keeping includes the use of film badges and dosimeters, monitoring of the laboratory area, waste disposal records, and adherence to local and federal laws.
- **What is a rad?**
  A rad, which stands for radiation absorbed dose, is the amount of radiation energy absorbed by a given biologic structure. It is used clinically to describe the amount of exposure to a given organ or organs of interest.

■ **What is a roentgen?**

A roentgen is a measure of gamma or x-ray radiation in air. It is used as the amount of exposure dose produced by a source.

■ **What is rem?**

Rem stands for roentgen equivalent man. It is the unit of human absorbed dose. It is used as the exposure value for monitoring devices as well as for the values for the recommended maximum permissible dose.

■ **What is a crystal scintillation counter?**

It is a thallium-activated sodium iodide crystal coupled to a photomultiplier tube. As energy photons enter the crystal and interact with the crystal molecules, minute flashes of light occur. These are detected and magnified by an electronic photomultiplier tube. The resultant electrical energy is amplified and proportionately counted.

■ **What is a liquid scintillation system?**

It is a detector system that measures the beta-producing radiation of a radionuclide dissolved in a liquid scintillation fluid.

■ **Describe a pulse height analyzer.**

Each radionuclide has a distinct energy spectrum. By electronic discrimination, either or both of the lower or higher energy ranges may be rejected, and a given radionuclide energy peak can be maximized for counting without interference by background counts or other radiation sources. The area between this lower threshold and upper threshold is called the "window."

■ **Describe a nuclide generator, or "cow."**

It consists of a shielded container in which there is a long-lived parent radionuclide that produces a short-lived daughter nuclide. This short-lived nuclide can be separated and used as needed. An example is molybdenum-99, which produces technetium-99M, having a 6-hour half-life. The technetium can be eluted from the parent molybdenum and used as needed.

■ **Describe the principle of competitive binding.**

Given a stoichiometric reversible reaction such as $Y + Z \leftrightarrows YZ$, the addition of more molecules of Y will result in a proportioned distribution of these new molecules of Y in the end product, YZ. This proportion of distribution is directly related to the concentration of YZ. That is, the greater the concentration of YZ, the more original Y molecules displaced by the new Y: $Y + Y^* + Z \leftrightarrows YZ + Y^*Z$. If these new molecules of Y can be identified with a radioactive label, and if the parent substance can be separated from the substrate, a value of displacement can be determined. By using a range of standards of YZ, a curve of concentration may be drawn and the concentration of the original substance can be determined.

■ **What is the principle of radioimmunoassay?**

Radioimmunoassay is a saturation and displacement analysis that is not unlike competitive binding but uses the antigen-antibody reaction rather than the binding protein as the receptor site. Antibody does not discriminate between labeled and unlabeled antigen. Hence, the addition of labeled antigen to a serum having an unknown amount of unlabeled antigen followed by a specific antibody will result in proportional distribution of labeled and unlabeled antigen bound to this antibody. If the amount of original unlabeled antigen is small, i.e., if the patient's serum level is low, proportionately greater amounts of labeled antigen will be bound to antibody and less unlabeled antigen will be free in the reaction mixture. The ratio of this bound to free radioactive antigen will be relatively high. If the patient's serum level is high, the ratio of bound to free radioactive antigen will be relatively smaller. Hence, the drawing of a standard curve using increasingly known concentrations of purified antigen allows this ratio of bound to free radionuclide to be expressed as a known value.

■ **What is the T3 test?**

Triiodothyronine, T3, is a physiologic precursor to thyroxine, T4. Thyroxine-binding globulin (TBG) preferentially binds T4 before T3. In the hyperthyroid state, the TBG is saturated with T4, and any exogenous radioactive T3 incubated with TBG will not be bound. In hypothyroid conditions, the TBG will take up the radioactive T3 since binding sites are available. After incubation, the unbound T3 is absorbed and counted. In hyperthyroidism, since there is more available unbound T3, the value obtained will be above the normal range. In hypothyroidism, the value obtained will be below the normal range. When the TBG level itself is elevated, especially by pregnancy and birth control medication, the number of binding sites is increased, allowing for increased absorption of radioactive T3 and less residual available for counting. This produces a spurious low count resembling hypothyroidism.

■ **What is the T4 test?**

Thyroxine (T4) is released from the patient's TBG by denaturation. This released T4 is incubated with exogenous TBG whose own T4 is labeled with radioactive iodine. In the principle of competitive binding, the original released T4 competes with the labeled T4. The amount of release of the labeled T4 is proportional to the number of original molecules of T4 in the patient. Physical separation extracts the unbound T4. Increased patient thyroxine results in the high release of radioactive counts in the extract and corresponds to hyperthyroidism. A low residual radioactive count indicates the low level of T4 in hypothyroidism. The specific assay value can be determined by forming a standard curve using purified thyroxine.

Increased TBG, as seen in pregnancy and contraceptive medication, results in spurious high counts and resembles hyperthryoidism.

■ **What is the T7 test value?**

It is a mathematical formulation using the T3 and T4 values in order to compensate for the high T4 and low T3 in pregnancy and contraceptive medication.

■ **What is the ETR?**

The effective thyroxine ratio (ETR) is a single in vitro procedure that considers the thyroid-binding globulin and total serum T4. It combines the competitive binding procedure of the T4 determination with a TBG absorption method analogous to the T3 procedure. It is unaffected by pregnancy or contraceptive medication.

■ **Describe the radioactive iodine uptake.**

The patient receives an oral dose of radioactive iodine. The number of radioactive counts taken over the neck is compared at a timed interval to the number of counts present in a standard geometric form containing an identical dose. The percent uptake is below normal in hypothyroidism or in previous high intake of iodine or x-ray dyes. The uptake is elevated in hyperthyroidism.

■ **Describe the principle of radioactive blood volume determination.**

A known amount of radioactive material is injected intravenously. A similar amount of radioactivity is diluted as a standard pool. After dilution in the patient, a blood sample is drawn and compared with an equivalent sample from the standard pool. The total circulating blood volume can then be mathematically extrapolated.

■ **What radionuclides may be used in determining blood volume?**

Many may be used. However, the radioactive iodinated serum albumin (RISA) labeled with ^{125}I is the most commonly used material.

■ **Can chromium 51 (^{51}Cr) be used for the determination of blood volume?**

Yes. ^{51}Cr labels the red cell. If washed labeled red cells are injected and recovered after equilibration in the patient, comparison to a pool standard and the use of the hematocrit can determine total blood volume.

■ **What is the ^{51}Cr red cell survival?**

^{51}Cr-labeled red cells are injected and sampled periodically over 2 to 3 weeks. The loss of radioactivity is compared with the known standard value curve. Rapid loss indicates bleeding or hemolysis.

■ **Describe the Schilling test.**

It is a test for the absorption of vitamin B_{12}. An oral dose of vitamin B_{12} labeled with radioactive cobalt is administered, followed by the collection of a 24-hour urine specimen. If there is reduced intestinal absorption of vitamin B_{12} or lack of gastric intrinsic factor, a small amount of radioactive vitamin B_{12} is recovered in the urine. In a repetition of the test with the addition of oral intrinsic factor (desiccated hog stomach), the patient whose absorption defect is a lack of his own intrinsic factor, as in pernicious anemia, will demonstrate more normal recovery of the radioactive material.

■ **Describe the plasma-iron clearance.**

^{59}Fe is injected into the patient. Blood samples are drawn at frequent timed intervals for 2 hours. The time of disappearance of the radioiron to half of the original is noted. This time is shortened in active marrow turnover conditions, such as iron deficiency or hemolytic anemia.

■ **Describe the plasma-iron turnover rate.**

Using the plasma-iron clearance, the total serum iron, and the total plasma volume, the rate of iron turnover can be determined by formula. This turnover is increased in active marrow turnover conditions, such as iron deficiency and hemolytic anemia.

■ **Describe red cell utilization.**

By using the same radioactive iron as that given for the plasma-iron clearance but by obtaining blood samples over a period of 2 weeks, the percent of the original dose absorbed by the red cells can be determined. This percentage is high and rapid in active marrow turnovers. It is low and slow in myelofibrosis and aplastic anemia.

■ **Describe the radioactive fat studies.**

A complete fat (triolein) labeled with radioactive iodine is given orally. If there is a fat-splitting pancreatic enzyme (lipase) present and if there is intestinal integrity, much of this fat will be absorbed. This level of absorption can be tested by collecting stool and determining the low level of residual radioactivity or by collecting blood and determining the elevated level of radioactivity over a period of 4 to 6 hours. If either lipase or intestinal integrity is impaired, the blood levels will be low and the stool levels will be high. To distinguish between the two possible deficiencies, the test is repeated using a fatty acid (oleic acid) labeled with radioactive iodine. This fatty acid does not require lipase for absorption. If the blood level remains low or the stool level high, poor intestinal integrity or malabsorption is indicated. If the blood level is high and the stool level is low in radioactivity, the indication is poor pancreatic function.

CHAPTER 6

Microbiology and immunology

Silas G. Farmer and Richard A. Komorowski

■ **What are the different sterilization methods commonly used in the laboratory? Name one application for each.**

Autoclaving, or moist heat under pressure (15 lbs, 15 minutes), is the best method of sterilization of materials that are not adversely affected by this treatment. Ethylene oxide sterilization is the method of choice for plastics and other solids that cannot withstand high heat. Filtration through membrane filters or fritted glass filters is to be used for sterilizing liquids such as carbohydrate solutions, serum, and urea solutions.

■ **What is meant by selective, differential, and enrichment media?**

A selective medium is one in which some agent has been added to offer a selective advantage to one or more organisms. Hence Thayer-Martin medium with VCN offers a selective advantage to *Neisseria gonorrhoeae* and *N. meningitidis,* because the antibiotics V (vancomycin), C (colistin), and N (nystatin) effectively inhibit most other *Neisseria* species as well as many other bacteria and yeast that may be found in reproductive cultures.

A differential medium permits the differentiation between two organisms with respect to one or more characteristics. For example, a simple carbohydrate such as glucose and an indicator that changes color after lowering the pH following growth permits the differentiation between those that can and those that cannot ferment (or oxidize) that carbohydrate.

An enrichment medium contains ingredients to enrich the formulation, usually to permit the isolation of the more fastidious microorganisms. Enrichments may be vitamins, yeast extract, serum, or other growth-stimulating components.

Media used in the clinical laboratory frequently contain one or more of the above characteristics. Hence, Thayer-Martin is both a selective medium because of the VCN and an enrichment medium because of the Iso-Vitalex additive.

■ **What is coagulase?**

Coagulase is a kinase produced by most pathogenic *Staphylococcus aureus*. If allowed to interact with a plasma factor (coagulase-reacting factor, or CRF), it will produce a thrombokinaselike active principle, which will convert fibrinogen into fibrin and result in clotting. However, unlike thrombokinase, the CRF does not require calcium for its formation. The extracellular coagulase, or "free coagulase," is best detected with rabbit plasma in a test tube.

The "bound coagulase," or clumping factor, does not require CRF, is performed as a slide test, and may be detected with human plasma.

Although good correlation is observed between the two methods, a negative slide test is best followed up with the tube test.

■ **What is ONPG and why is it used?**

ONPG is o-nitrophenyl-β-D-galactopyranoside and is the reagent used to detect the enzyme β-galactosidase.

Lactose fermentation requires the presence of β-galactosidase, an intracellular enzyme, and a permease. In the absence of permease, potentially lactose-fermenting organisms are unable to do so because of the inability of the lactose to enter the cell. In the ONPG test, the organisms are grown on a lactose-containing medium that encourages the development of β-galactoside permease mutants. Thus, the presence of potential lactose fermenters, which otherwise might be considered as late fermenters or even nonfermenters, may be detected. In the positive test, β-galactosidase splits o-nitrophenol, a yellow compound, from ONPG.

Although not recommended as a substitute for the lactose fermentation test, the ONPG test is nevertheless useful in detecting late lactose-fermenting *E. coli*, *Klebsiella*, and other members of the Enterobacteriaceae family. Another useful application is in differentiating Salmonella (ONPG negative) from *Citrobacter* and *Arizona* organisms (both ONPG positive).

■ **What enzyme is produced by an indole-positive organism and how is it detected?**

Tryptophanase is detected by means of the widely used procedure known as Kovac's method. The reagent is prepared by dissolving p-dimethylaminobenzaldehyde in amyl or isoamyl alcohol, which is then acidified with concentrated HCl. When this reagent is added to a culture containing indole, a deep red color develops.

■ **What portion of the pneumococcus is associated with virulence?**

In the mouse model, the presence of the capsule has been shown to be the virulence factor. A few encapsulated pneumococci will produce a fatal disease, whereas as many as 1×10^6 nonencapsulated ones (derived from the same serotype) will not.

In man, phagocytosis is retarded by the presence of a capsule. The virulence factors are poorly understood, but one is thought to be a neuraminidase.

■ **What differences exist between alpha and beta hemolysis other than the color surrounding the colony?**

Beta hemolysis is characterized by complete hemolysis of RBCs surrounding the colony. The two hemolysins are oxygen-labile streptolysin O and oxygen-stable streptolysin S. Although only streptolysin S produces hemolysis around surface colonies, both O and S produce hemolysis in the deep-cut section of the blood agar or in the test tube suspension of RBCs.

The alpha-hemolytic streptococci are surrounded by a narrow zone of incomplete hemolysis in which unhemolyzed RBCs adjacent to the colony may be seen microscopically. This zone may be surrounded by a zone of complete hemolysis. Because of the formation of an unidentified reductant of hemoglobin, green discoloration of the medium surrounding the colony may occur with some species of RBCs under certain conditions of incubation.

■ **Explain the meaning and processing of a blood agar plate with beta hemolysis only in the cut portion.**

The most probable explanation is that the organism is a beta-hemolytic streptococcus that is producing only streptolysin O and not streptolysin S. The specimen should be handled in the same manner as any other beta-hemolytic streptococcus.

■ **Why is it clinically useful to group beta-hemolytic streptocci?**

Beta-hemolytic streptococci represent a very heterogeneous group with diverse clinical significance. The most important is group A in causing human disase. Recently, group B has been increasingly associated with neonatal and adult infection. Some members of group D compose the enterococci. The clinical significance of other groups varies greatly. Although group A streptococci are exquisitely sensitive to penicillin, some other streptococci are quite different in their antibiotic susceptibility.

■ **Which serotypes of group A** *Streptococcus pyogenes* **are associated with acute glomerulonephritis?**

M protein types 4, 12, 25, and 49 have the greatest association, although occasionally a new M type has been described.

■ **Which streptococci are of increasing concern in neonatal infection?**

Streptococcus agalactiae, or group B of the Lancefield classification, is significant in neonatal infection.

■ **What are enterococci and why is it clinically important to identify these organisms?**

Enterococci are enteric streptococci belonging to the Lancefield group D. *S. faecalis, S. faecalis* var. *liquefaciens,* and *S. faecium* are nonhemolytic, but *S. faecalis* var. *zymogenes* and *S. durans* produce beta hemolysis on blood agar. Some members of the serologic group D are not enterococci, e.g., *S. bovis* and *S. equinus.*

The enterococci are not as sensitive to penicillin as the group A streptococci. The antibiotic dosage must be adjusted upward to effectively treat infections caused by the enterococci, e.g., endocarditis.

■ **What test can be used in the laboratory to differentiate between streptococci and staphylococci?**

Catalase is the test of choice. The staphylococci and micrococci produce catalase, which is easily detected by adding a drop of 3% hydrogen peroxide to the bacteria and observing bubble formation. Inasmuch as blood contains small amounts of catalase, care must be exercised when testing organisms growing on blood agar.

■ **Differentiate between** *Edwardsiella tarda, Arizona hinshawii, Citrobacter freundii,* **and most** *Salmonella* **organisms.**

Citrobacter differs from the rest of these organisms in that it lacks lysine decarboxylase. Of the remaining, *E. tarda* differs from the *Arizona* and *Salmonella* organisms by being indole positive. A positive malonate differentiates the *Arizona* from the *Salmonella* organisms. Of course, the latter two could be differentiated on a serologic basis.

■ **Are members of the family Enterobacteriaceae only enteric pathogens?**

No. Some members are plant pathogens, and some produce infection only when found outside of the gut. The most significant enteric pathogens are *Salmonella, Shigella,* enteropathogenic *E. coli,* and *Yersinia enterocolitica.* The recent inclusion of *Yersinia* in the family brings along *Y. pestis (Pasteurella pestis)* and adds a whole new dimension to the clinical syndromes associated with this family.

■ **The biochemical reactions of an enteric organism are as follows: negative reactions for phenylalanine deaminase, H_2S, gas from glucose, lysine decarboxylase, lactose fermentation, citrate utilization, and malonate. It is positive for ornithine decarboxylase and urease and is motile at 25° C. What might the organism be and of what clinical significance is this organism?**

An aerogenic, lactose-negative, urease-producing gram-negative bacillus that is motile only at 25° C is very suggestive of *Yersinia enterocolitica*. *Yersinia* produce mainly enteric syndromes such as cervical adenitis, enteritis, enterocolitis, terminal ileitis, appendicitis, and diarrhea. Occasionally, cases of septicemia and, even less often, cases of meningitis have been observed.

■ **What is the clinical importance of *Pseudomonas aeruginosa*?**

Members of the genus *Pseudomonas* are widespread in nature and usually cause little concern for the healthy individual. In the burn patient, *P. aeruginosa* rapidly colonizes the eschar because of antibiotic therapy used to suppress the staphylococci, and this frequently leads to fatal infection. Nosocomial infections, especially pulmonary disease in patients on respiration equipment for extended periods of time and renal disease in patients who have had instrumentation, continue to cause concern to infectious disease control committees in hospitals.

■ **Which anaerobe produces a black pigment and what is the clinical significance of this organism?**

Bacteroides melaninogenicus produces a black pigment. It has been associated with infections of the female genital tract, bone and joint infections, liver and pulmonary abscesses, intestinal lesions, and infections of the mouth and gums.

■ **What differences are noted between *Mycobacterium tuberculosis* and *M. kansasii*?**

M. tuberculosis usually appears as a dry, colorless to buff colony on inspissated egg media and is characterized by production of niacin and reduction of nitrates to nitrites.

Although *M. kansasii* is usually buff-colored when first seen, it is photochromogenic, producing a yellow color after exposure to light and continued incubation. The colony is usually smooth and is characterized by no niacin production and by reduction of nitrates. It must be recalled that some strains of *M. tuberculosis* that are resistant to isoniazid (INH) may be unable to produce niacin.

■ **Is *Mycobacterium tuberculosis* resistant to heat?**

Although *M. tuberculosis* may remain viable in culture media and dried sputum for up to 8 months and is quite resistant to chemical disinfection, it is as sensitive to moist heat as are other vegetative forms of bacteria. Therefore, pasteurization temperatures are effective in eliminating the tubercle bacillus from milk and milk products.

■ **What are L-forms and how may they be cultivated?**

L-forms are cell wall–deficient (CWD) forms of bacteria that may be induced by antibiotics that act on cell wall synthesis (such as penicillin) and complement, for example. They are osmotically fragile and can survive and reproduce only in a hypertonic environment.

Nutritional media adequate to support the parental type of the species and containing 0.3 mole sucrose or 20% serum will usually grow most L-forms.

■ **What is the clinical significance of CWD- or L-forms?**

Although CWD- or L-forms are not capable of producing disease, they may revert back to the parental type on removal from the environment that induced them (i.e., discontinuing the antibiotic therapy), with the resulting virulence and pathogenicity of the parental type.

■ **How can *Mycoplasma pneumoniae* be isolated?**

Mycoplasma organisms are really bacteria without cell walls and therefore must be cultivated in a hypertonic medium. The use of PPLO medium base enriched with 20% serum, yeast extract, and agents to restrict the growth of other oral and pharyngeal organisms (e.g., penicillin, amphotericin B, and thallium acetate) will usually suffice. An aerobic atmosphere is preferable. Inasmuch as 7 to 9 days may be required for isolation, plates must be taped to prevent desiccation during the incubation.

■ **In what ways can disease-producing microorganisms be transmitted?**

In 1535 Fracastorius de Verona said that the seeds of disease could be transmitted (1) by direct contact, (2) by fomites, and (3) ad distans, or at great distances, via aerosol. He was right! We have added new vehicles, such as frozen foods, transfused blood, and venipuncture needles, but we have not added to the basic understanding of disease transmission.

■ **What organisms may cause food poisoning?**

Food poisoning may be caused by *Clostridium botulinum* and *Staphylococcus aureus*. In food poisoning, the viable organism need not be present to produce the toxicosis.

■ **What is food infection?**

Food infection is a gastrointestinal disease caused by the ingestion

of rather large numbers of viable bacteria in food. This type of disorder may be found with *Salmonella, Clostridium perfringens,
Shigella,* and *Vibrio parahaemolyticus.* In contrast, food poisoning
caused by *C. botulinum* or *S. aureus* does not require the ingestion of
viable bacteria but just their toxins and thus is a primary toxicosis.

■ **What is the difference between bacteremia and septicemia?**

Bacteremia merely designates the presence of bacteria in the
bloodstream. This may be a simple transient bacteremia following a
vigorous tooth brushing or a signifiant one leading to symptoms of
sepsis. Septicemia implies disease and therefore symptoms (fever,
toxic reactions with or without shock, and so on).

■ **What guidelines are reasonable to follow in the collection of blood
cultures with respect to the number, timing, and so on?**

Blood cultures are indicated in the febrile patient during the actual
fever. Most organisms may be recovered from the bloodstream at any
time during the bacteremia. However, some, such as *Brucella,* tend
to be tissue parasites and are shed periodically. For this reason, several blood cultures should be drawn.

The most reasonable guidelines suggest a routine of three blood
cultures drawn over the period of 1 working day. More frequent blood
cultures over a longer period of time may be required if brucellosis is
suspected.

■ **What is Liquoid, or SPS, and what effects does it exert in the
blood culture?**

Liquoid, or SPS, is sodium polyanethol sulfonate. It is an anticoagulant of much less toxicity than oxalate or citrate; when incorporated into blood culture broth at a final concentration of 0.05%, it is an-
ticomplementary and inhibits both the bactericidal action of blood
and the phagocytic activity of leukocytes. Bacteria survive more readily in Liquoid than in citrated blood and are more readily recovered in
broth cultures.

■ **What visible signs are suggestive of bacterial growth in a blood culture bottle? How would you handle a bottle that did not display
these signs?**

Turbidity in the supernate, white colonies lying on top of the
sedimented cells, and early hemolysis are all suggestive of bacterial
growth. However, *Brucella, Neisseria meningitidis, Haemophilus influenzae,* yeast, and others may not produce sufficient growth (greater
than 1×10^6 organisms/ml) to produce turbidity.

Bottles that do not show the above characteristics should be subcultured to enriched agar at 24 or 48 hours and again before discarding as "no growth" to detect positive cultures that are not grossly apparent.

■ **What bacteria may be isolated from blood cultures?**

Almost any bacterium may be isolated from blood cultures. Some of the isolates may be virulent pathogens such as *Staphylococcus aureus, Escherichia coli, Proteus,* or others capable of producing sepsis in any individual. Others may be low-grade pathogens that usually infect only the compromised host, such as *Staphylococcus epidermidis, Flavobacterium,* or *Citrobacter freundii.* Some isolates may represent only the indigenous flora of the skin and not a bacteremia. This may result from inadequate preparation of the skin before collection of the specimen.

■ **What explanation might be offered for the frequent isolation of low-grade pathogens, or opportunists, from blood culture bottles?**

Organisms that make up the indigenous flora of the skin (e.g., *Staphylococcus epidermidis* and diphtheroids) are frequently recovered from the blood culture bottle because the venipuncture site was not properly disinfected.

■ **A patient is suspected of having typhoid fever. What specimens, taken at what times, are indicated for laboratory analysis?**

During the first week, most patients have septicemia, and a positive blood culture may be obtained. About 25% of these patients will also have a positive urine culture during this time. Positive stool cultures may be obtained about the second week of illness, and at about that time agglutinins appear in the serum. A second agglutination titer should be obtained about 10 days to 2 weeks after the first in order to demonstrate a fourfold or greater increase in titer.

Of course, not all of these procedures may be required. A positive blood culture would suffice. However, if the blood culture is negative or if the patient has passed that phase of illness in which septicemia is a component, the other procedures would be indicated.

■ **Anaerobic bacteria may cause serious pulmonary infection. Which specimens are acceptable and which are not acceptable for anaerobic culture?**

A transtracheal aspirate is the only specimen that can produce meaningful clinical results as of this date. Potentially, the bronchial brush technique may offer good specimens. Sputum or bronchial washings are invariably contaminated with the indigenous anaerobic oral flora and are not acceptable for anaerobic culture.

■ **What are the best methods for the digestion and processing of sputum cultures for *Mycobacterium tuberculosis*?**

Sodium hydroxide and trisodium phosphate were used for many years to digest the mucus and decontaminate the specimen. However, the best method is the use of NAC (*N*-acetyl-L-cysteine) and sodium hydroxide.

■ **Discuss how you would handle a cloudy spinal fluid in the microbiology laboratory.**

Any spinal fluid with an abnormal white blood count should be processed promptly. A gram-stained smear should be made of the sediment, and if bacteria are seen the results should be reported immediately to the physician. If bacteria are present, the choice of media is more apparent. However, if cultures are to be set up without this knowledge, inoculate media that would support the growth of *N. meningitidis*, pneumococcus, *H. influenzae*, and streptococci. A blood agar and chocolate agar with enrichment incubated at 35° to 37° C in 5% to 10% CO_2 should suffice.

Cultures for fungi or *M. tuberculosis* are usually not performed unless specifically requested.

■ **Which is the better atmosphere for incubating blood agar plates from respiratory cultures, O_2 or CO_2?**

Carbon dioxide is preferable for several reasons. Some pneumococcal strains are capnophilic (require CO_2) and would be missed if not grown in that atmosphere.

■ **What organisms are most frequently associated with primary urinary tract infection in the female?**

Usually *E. coli* (85%), because of the shortness of the female urethra and the anatomic proximity to the fecal flora.

■ **A gram-stained smear of exudate from a cervicofacial draining nodule reveals gram-positive branching filaments. What clinical diagnosis is suggested?**

A clinical diagnosis of actinomycosis is suggested. *Actinomyces israelii* and *A. naeslundii* are the two most frequently encountered species.

■ **Trench mouth, or Vincent's angina, is a fusospirochetal symbiotic disease. How would you process a request and what would you look for? What is the limitation of the procedure?**

A smear from the diseased portion stained with Wright's, carbolfuchsin, or some other strong stain and examined for fusiform bacilli and *Borrelia* is the proper procedure. Inasmuch as the organisms that cause Vincent's angina are indigenous oral flora, they are of significance only when they are present in large numbers.

An alternative method of examination would be to make a hanging-drop examination from the affected area and view with a dark field. *Treponema microdentium* would also be seen by this method.

The diagnosis of Vincent's angina is a clinical one and cannot be made by the laboratory solely on the basis of examination of the smears.

■ **What are some frequent causes of bacterial pneumonia in the adult?**

Streptococcus (Diplococcus) pneumoniae continues to be the most frequently encountered species, occuring in about 75% of the patients. About 10% are caused by various gram-negative bacilli of the family Enterobacteriaceae (e.g., *Klebsiella pneumoniae, E. coli, Enterobacter*) and about 7% are staphylococcal in origin. The rest may be *Haemophilus influenzae, Mycoplasma pneumoniae,* or anaerobic gram-negative bacilli.

■ **What is the significance of many epithelial cells in a smear from a specimen labeled "sputum"?**

The presence of many epithelial cells indicates that the specimen was contaminated with salvia and is therefore an improper specimen for processing. The bacteria encountered represent the indigenous oral flora rather than the organisms involved in the patient's respiratory tract infection. The simple expedient of rinsing the mouth before sputum collection will do much to remove the saliva contamination. However, the transtracheal aspiration is bacteriologically the best technique for processing.

■ **Describe proper collection and examination technique for the flagellated protozoon that causes a venereal disease.**

Trichomonas vaginalis is the only trichomonad found in the vagina or the urethral tract. Diagnosis may be made by preparing saline wet mounts of vaginal exudate and examining with the microscope. The typical nervous, jerky, trichomonal movement and the characteristic undulating membrane readily identify this protozoon. Some authors have reported better luck with culture techniques, however.

■ **Describe a positive smear for gonorrhea in a male with acute urethritis.**

Uncomplicated gonorrhea in the male is characterized by acute urethritis with a marked purulent reaction. A gram-stained smear would reveal many polymorphonuclear leukocytes (PMNs) with many intracellular and extracellular gram-negative diplococci. Although this is the typical picture, the organism *Neisseria gonorrhoeae* cannot be legally identified by smear alone. The report of the smear should contain. the observation but should also contain the phrase: "which is morphologically similar to *N. gonorrhoeae.*"

■ **Why is it not a good idea to diagnose gonorrhea from a cervical or vaginal smear?**

Many bacteria may be seen on smears from these areas and some of the gram-negative bacilli may resemble *N. gonorrhoeae* morphologically. In addition, many women are asymptomatic and have *N. gonorrhoeae* present in low numbers. Culture of multiple sites, such as cervical, anal, vaginal, and pharyngeal areas, is necessary to detect all cases of gonorrhea.

■ **What bacteria would you normally expect to find in the vagina?**

Women of childbearing age might have *Lactobacillus, Corynebacterium, Staphylococcus, Micrococcus,* streptococci (beta-hemolytic *S. faecalis,* other aerobic streptococci, and *Peptostreptococcus*), *E. coli, Proteus, Candida,* and *Clostridium perfringens.*

■ **A patient is seen with a shallow ulcer on his penis and swollen lymph nodes or buboes. What infections might this suggest?**

This might be lymphogranuloma venereum, granuloma inguinale, or chancroid.

■ **What precautions should be followed in preparing slide mounts of fungi that have a white aerial mycelium?**

Many laboratory contaminants, dermatophytes, and systemic fungi are characterized by white aerial mycelium. Inasmuch as the identity of the fungus cannot be ascertained with accuracy by the gross appearance of the mycelium, it is best to handle all specimens as if they were highly infectious. The use of laminar flow hoods and the practice of "wetting down" the aerial mycelium by carefully overlaying the slant with sterile water or saline solution should be practiced. The distribution of aerial spores is to be avoided. Although the distribution of contaminant spores creates only laboratory contamination, the spores of *Coccidioides immitis, Blastomyces dermatitidis,* and *Histoplasma capsulatum* are highly infectious to laboratory personnel.

■ **What methods may be used to quantitate gentamycin?**

The classic tube dilution method is not adequate for the assay of gentamycin because it requires too much time (18 to 24 hours) and is not sensitive enough (serial twofold decrements) for the clinical evaluation of patients.

A rapid (3- to 4-hour) procedure by Sabath, which measures the ability of gentamycin (or any other aminoglycoside) to inhibit the germination of *Bacillus subtilis* spores, is reproducible within ±10% and results are available before the next scheduled dose of antibiotic. This procedure is easily performed even in the small clinical laboratory, and the plates used in the assay may be stored in the refrigerator for several weeks. The most recent method available for the assay of gentamycin, and one that overcomes the problem inherent in the situation in which the patient is taking several antibiotics, is a sensitive, specific, and rapid method that requires minute amounts of serum. R factor–mediated enzymes that adenylate or acetylate gentamycin have been employed in a radioactive assay. ATP serves as the source for the adenyl group (or acetyl-CoA for the acetyl group) that is transferred to the antibiotic during the reaction. Adenylated or acetylated gentamycin, but not ATP, is positively charged and therefore binds to the negatively charged phosphocellulose (PC) paper. When aliquots of the mixture containing ^{14}C-ATP are pipetted onto PC paper and washed to eliminate nonspecifically bound radioactivity, the PC-bound radioactivity measures adenylated or acetylated antibiotic.

The RIA procedure may also be used to quantitate this antibiotic.

■ **What is the clinical usefulness of a serum gentamycin assay?**

Gentamycin is relatively toxic. It causes ototoxicity in approximately 2.3% of patients but renal damage in fewer patients. The ototoxicity is usually correlated with previous otologic status, prior therapy with other ototoxic drugs, age, and the serum concentrations. However, since gentamycin is excreted primarily by the kidneys, serum concentrations reflect the dosage, route of administration, interval between doses, and renal function of the patient.

Most dosage schedules aim to attain a concentration of about 4μg/ml gentamycin in serum. However, concentrations above 10 to 12μg/ml are considered potentially toxic.

Although serum concentration correlates with renal function, the half-life cannot be calculated from creatinine clearance or serum creatinine concentrations in the acutely ill or dehydrated individual or in one who has minimal muscle mass. Thus, a rapid and accurate serum assay is needed to avoid toxic levels of gentamycin.

■ **What do the terms MIC and MBC designate and of what clinical use are they?**

They represent minimum inhibitory concentration (MIC) and minimum bactericidal concentration (MBC). They are usually used to designate the concentration of antibiotic that is required to inhibit or kill an organism. This information is useful in initiating or quantitating antibiotic therapy, especially if the treatment is to be given over a protracted period.

■ **Discuss the principle, procedure, and value of the Schlicter test.**

The Schlicter test is a twofold tube dilution test to determine the total killing power of the serum against the organism causing the patient's infection. This test measures the effects of one or more antibiotics, complement, or other "cidal" agents in the patient's serum. A cidal effect at a serum dilution of fourfold is acceptable, but an eightfold cidal titer is preferable.

Those tubes in which no visible growth is observed should be subcultured to antibiotic-free media to ascertain whether the organisms have been killed or were only inhibited. The results can be expressed as the bacteriostatic titer (highest serum dilution that inhibits growth) and the bactericidal titer (highest serum dilution that kills the organism).

■ **Which organisms cannot be tested for antibiotic susceptibility by the Kirby-Bauer disc diffusion method?**

The Kirby-Bauer test was devised for the rapidly growing aerobic bacteria. This procedure cannot be used for slow-growing bacteria such as *M. tuberculosis* or any of the anaerobic bacteria. Atmospheres such as carbon dioxide change the pH of the medium to acid and affect the action of some antibiotics.

■ **What variables might influence the zone size in the Kirby-Bauer antibiotic sensitivity test?**

Possible sources of variability include the age and size of the inoculum, the manner in which the plate is inoculated, the antibiotic content of the disc, medium concentration, pH, moisture content of agar, thickness of agar, length of incubation, method of illuminating, and reading zones.

■ **What is the usefulness of the Maloney test?**

The Maloney test is used to detect hypersensitivity to the diphtheria toxoid. It is used in the adult to prevent anaphylactic shock after administration of the toxoid.

■ **What is the Schick test?**

The Schick test is an intradermal skin test used to detect the presence of circulating antibodies to the diphtheria toxin. Although not correlated 100% with immunity, for practical purposes it is usually assumed that if no redness and induration appear after the injection of 0.1 ml containing $1/50$ minimum lethal dose (MLD), the individual has

$1/500$ to $1/250$ unit of antitoxin/ml and thus is protected against the toxic action of the diphtheria bacillus.

■ **What is the Neufeld-Quellung reaction and to which organisms may it be applied?**

The Neufeld-Quellung reaction is a swelling of the polysaccharide capsular material in the presence of homologous antibody. Any organism with a capsular polysaccharide may demonstrate this reaction. *Streptococcus (Diplococcus) pneumoniae, Klebsiella,* and *Haemophilus* are frequently typed by this procedure.

■ **What is the purpose of heating the bacterial suspension when performing some agglutination reactions with the Salmonelleae?**

Some *Salmonella* organisms contain a Vi antigen, which is an envelope antigen that, if present in sufficient amount, can mask the detection of the underlying somatic, or O, antigens. These envelope antigens are thermolabile and thus are destroyed by heat to reveal the O antigens. It is a good practice to test the bacterial suspension with anti-Vi antiserum.

■ **What is the value of quality control in microbiology?**

Quality control means that all the factors that are important for the accurate analysis are known to be performing properly. The specimen has been properly collected, correctly processed, and plated on media that will support characteristic growth in a known environment. The personnel can recognize the growth and identify the significant isolate with media and reagents that are known to give accurate results. The report is transmitted to proper recording areas without error. In general, you are confident that the analysis has been correct and complete.

■ **Many laboratories use TSI, KIA, or RDS for enteric bacteriology. What is the meaning of "acid/acid," "alk/acid," etc. on these media?**

These media are characterized by the incorporation of two or three carbohydrates in different concentrations in an agar slant containing an indicator. Usually glucose is present in 0.1% concentration and lactose or lactose and sucrose in 1.0% concentrations.

The slant represents aerobic growth conditions, whereas the butt is more anaerobic. If only the CHO present in low concentration (i.e., glucose in the above examples) was fermented, the entire tube would become acid (yellow with a phenol red indicator) initially, but in the aerobic slant the reaction would proceed to completion through the Krebs' cycle to form CO_2 and water. At this time (24 hours), the slant would appear to be unchanged (it would appear red or alkaline). The butt, lacking oxygen, could not pass beyond lactic acid or pyruvic acid, and the butt portion would be acid (yellow) because of the accumulation of the intermediary organic acids resulting from the degradation or fermentation of the CHO.

However, if the CHO present in greater concentration (1.0%— lactose and/or sucrose) was fermented, the reaction in the slant portion could not proceed to completion for several days and therefore would appear yellow, as would the butt.

■ **How could you isolate and identify pathogenic *Neisseria* from the upper respiratory tract?**

The two most important *Neisseria* in the upper respiratory tract are *Neisseria meningitidis* and *N. gonorrhoeae*. *N. gonorrhoeae* may produce gonococcal pharyngitis, and *N. meningitidis* may produce local inflammation of the pharynx before any central nervous system involvement or bacteremia. Both organisms will grow readily on Thayer-Martin medium with Iso-Vitalex enrichment and containing VCN in an atmosphere of 5% to 10% carbon dioxide at 35° to 37° C.

■ **What is the significance of a colony count of urine?**

It has been determined that rather low counts (organisms/ml) may be found under normal conditions and represent contamination of the urethra with indigenous flora. However, counts of 10^5/ml and greater are usually significant, indicating either current infection or a propensity to infectious sequelae, such as pyelonephritis, if the patient is asymptomatic.

■ **How would you culture a stool specimen from a patient with suspected bacterial diarrhea if there were no history of consumption of raw clams or travel to "cholera countries"?**

Promptness in processing is indicated. Make a suspension of the stool specimen in sterile saline solution and inoculate agar plates of MacConkey's brilliant green, XLD, Salmonella-Shigella, Hektoen, or other appropriate formulations. Inoculate gram-negative broth with part of the stool specimen for enrichment, and subculture to appropriate media after overnight incubation.

Colonies resembling *Salmonella, Shigella,* and enteropathogenic *E. coli* (if from a child) should be picked and inoculated onto differential media for biochemical identification and serologic typing, if indicated.

■ **Name several commonly encountered bacteria from spinal fluid and the age groups associated with each.**

Neisseria meningitidis causes a rather severe meningitis, worldwide in distribution, which occurs in both sporadic and epidemic forms. Although all ages may be involved, cases are more frequently seen among infants and young children. The disease is endemic in large cities, and epidemic periods may be seen in this country that coincide with major population movement and recruit training camps. In one reported series of 258 cases over a 3-year period, 48% occurred between the ages of 0 and 4 years, 17% between 5 and 14, 14% between 15 and 29, and the remaining 23% from age 30 or more.

Haemophilus influenzae is the most common form of suppurative meningitis between the neonatal period and age 6, the period when *N. meningitidis* is not epidemic. *H. influenzae* is the most common cause of bacterial meningitis. About 40% of the cases of *H. influenzae* meningitis occur before age 1 and another 53% between 1 and 4 years of age. The rest (7%) are scattered over the remaining years.

Pneumococcal meningitis is the third most common variety of acute bacterial meningitis. It is seen more commonly among infants and the elderly.

If one looks at neonatal meningitis, one sees a variety of bacterial causes. In one study of 94 cases in Los Angeles, during a 6-year period no bacteria were isolated and identified in 22 of the cases. In decreasing order of occurrence the identified species were *E. coli*, unidentified gram-negative bacilli of the family Enterobacteriaceae designated *Paracolon* (12), *Klebsiella* or *Enterobacter* (10), *Streptococcus* (8), *Proteus* (5), *Listeria monocytogenes* (5), *Salmonella* (3), *Staphylococcus epidermidis* (3), *Diplococcus pneumoniae* (2), *Haemophilus influenzae* (2), and *Pseudomonas* and Mimeae 1 each. Thus, in this study of meningitis in the neonate, of the bacteria isolated, more than 70% of the cases belong to the family Enterobacteriaceae.

■ **What is meant by "redox" potential and of what use is it in the laboratory?**

Redox potential is a term used to express the oxidation-reduction potential, or Eh (expressed as positive or negative millivolts), of the environment. The milieu of man varies greatly with respect to its Eh. Normal tissue has an Eh of about $+120$ mV, whereas the Eh of pus is about -230 mV. For reference, the Eh of hydrogen is -420 mV.

Organisms vary greatly in their aerotolerance; thus, aerobes such as *Pseudomonas* will not grow in a medium with a very low Eh. At the other end of the spectrum, strict anaerobes such as *Clostridium tetani* will not grow and sporulate if the Eh is too high. Most organisms, although they are considered aerobes, will also grow at very low Eh values and thus are termed facultative.

When one desires to isolate strict anaerobes from an abscess, one should select the conditions that give a very low Eh value, such as prereduced anaerobically sterilized (PRAS) medium with an Eh of about -150 mV. The pH of the medium will greatly influence the Eh value. The Eh value will become 60 mV more negative for each unit increase in the pH. Thus, a medium with an Eh value of $+100$ mV at pH 6 would have Eh values of $+40$ and -20 mV at pH values of 7 and 8, respectively.

■ **How does the Gas-Pak hydrogen-CO_2 generator work?**

Gas-Pak (BBL) is a commercially available envelope containing a hydrogen-producing sodium borohydride tablet and a citric acid + sodium bicarbonate tablet, which produces carbon dioxide. It is activated by adding 10 ml of water. A catalyst, active at room temperature, consists of alumina pellets coated with 0.5% palladium. Free molecular oxygen is thus combined with the hydrogen to form water and reduce the redox potential of the atmosphere sufficiently to support those organisms termed "anaerobes."

■ **What genera compose the family Enterobacteriaceae?**

Escherichia, Edwardsiella, Salmonella, Arizona, Shigella, Citrobacter, Klebsiella, Enterobacter, Serratia, Proteus, Providencia, Yersinia, and *Pectobacterium* compose the Enterobacteriaceae.

■ **What is the laboratory importance of bacterial dissociation?**

Most bacterial dissociation is of the S-R type (smooth to rough), with the resulting loss of superficial antigens. When these are necessary for antigenic analysis (i.e., typhoid bacillus or other Enterobacteriaceae agglutination, fluorescent antibody identification of *Bordetella pertussis,* or capsular typing of pneumococci), it is impossible to demonstrate the expected antigen-antibody reaction. Inasmuch as the S-R dissociation is usually not complete, it may be reversed by animal passage. For example, when a mixture of S and R forms is injected into an animal, the R (rough) forms are rapidly phagocytized and the S (smooth, virulent) forms persist and can be isolated.

■ **What effect does contaminating saliva have on the microbial content of sputum?**

Many organisms are found as indigenous oral flora and can be recovered from saliva. Many of these may represent only the transient flora. However, it is difficult to impossible to assign a role to many of the organisms solely on the basis of identification. Thus, a *Klebsiella pneumoniae* from saliva has the same characteristics as a *Klebsiella pneumoniae* from lobar pneumonia. Of significance also is the fact that some enzymes in saliva will mask the detection of or will lyse some bacteria such as *Streptococcus (Diplococcus) pneumoniae*.

■ **What effect does storage at room temperature for 4 or more hours have on the microbial content of sputum?**

The concentration of contaminating or nonpathogenic *Staphylococcus epidermidis, Neisseria* sp., *Streptococcus viridans*, and potentially pathogenic *Streptococcus pneumoniae, Haemophilus influenzae, Klebsiella, Enterobacter*, and *E. coli* increases 1 to 3 logs/ml after storage at room temperature for 4 or more hours. The concentration of some potential pathogens changes from a clinically insignificant 1×10^3 to a significant 1×10^6 or more organisms/ml.

■ **What test is useful to differentiate the *Proteus* and *Providencia* from other members of the family Enterobacteriaceae and from each other?**

Both *Proteus* and *Providencia* elaborate the enzyme phenylalanine or tryptophane deaminase and thus are separated from most of the other members of this family. They may be differentiated from one another by the urease test; the *Providencia* lack this enzyme.

Although some strains of *Enterobacter agglomerans* may produce a phenylalanine deaminase, they may be differentiated from these two genera by fermenting arabinose and being yellow (75%).

■ **How do endotoxins differ from exotoxins?**

Most exotoxins are readily released into the substrate, quite specific in their action, very antigenic, readily neutralized by their homologous antibody, and thermolabile. A notable exception is the thermostable enterotoxin of *Staphylococcus aureus*, the exotoxin that causes staphylococcal food poisoning.

Toxins, which are termed endotoxins, are very similar to each other in their action regardless of bacterial origin. They are weakly antigenic, not readily released from the bacterial cell, relatively heat stable, and produced primarily by gram-negative bacilli. Endotoxins are less toxic than exotoxins but if administered in sufficient quantity can cause fever and irreversible shock and exert an effect on nonspecific immunity.

■ **In what manner are the enterotoxins of *Staphylococcus aureus* different from other exotoxins?**

There are five emetic toxins produced by certain strains of *S. aureus* that are thermostable. They will survive heating to 100° C for 30 minutes. Another way to visualize this resistance to heat is to consider a chocolate eclair filled with custard and staphylococci (with one of the enterotoxins) after boiling for half an hour. You can imagine the appearance of the eclair—but the enterotoxins will still be present and active.

■ **What organisms may cause "gas" production with necrosis of tissue?**

The gas gangrene group of *Clostridia* such as *C. perfringens, C. septicum, C. novyi, C. histolyticum,* and *C. bifermentans.* In addition, members of the Enterobacteriaceae, such as *E. coli,* may be included. A gassy necrotic cellulitis caused by anaerobes or symbiotic action of *Peptostreptococcus* and *Staphylococcus aureus* may also be encountered.

■ **What two species of *Corynebacterium* elaborate a diphtheria toxin and how may they be differentiated?**

Corynebacterium diphtheriae, var. *mitis, gravis,* and *intermedius,* and *C. ulcerans* elaborate a diphtheria toxin. Pleomorphism is more pronounced in *C. ulcerans;* it does not reduce nitrates to nitrites, but it hydrolyzes urea and slowly liquefies gelatin.

■ **What is lockjaw and how can it be prevented?**

Lockjaw is one of the clinical manifestations of tetanus, which is an intoxication with the exotoxin of *Clostridium tetani.* It is characterized by intense, severe muscle spasms. The toxin, known as tetanospasmin, is among the most potent bacterial toxins known. Spores of *C. tetani* are introduced by contamination of a wound. The transformation of spores into toxin-producing vegetative forms requires a lower redox (oxidation-reduction) potential than is present in normal tissues. Necrosis resulting from the trauma or the presence of other bacteria can lower the redox potential sufficiently. The organism has little or no invasive capacity, but the toxin is absorbed into the CNS, bloodstream, and muscles. The major clinical manifestation of tetanus is muscular rigidity; when this involves the facial or masseter muscles, it is referred to as lockjaw or trismus. However, the toxicity will usually progress to general tetanus and cause violent contractions of the neck, trunk, and limb muscles.

Clinical tetanus is preventable by immunization with tetanus toxoid.

■ **Differentiate among the genera *Listeria, Erysipelothrix,* and *Corynebacterium.***

The organisms of all three of these genera are gram-positive bacilli and to the average person could not be differentiated on a morphologic basis.

E. rhusiopathiae can be separated from the catalase-negative *C. pyogenes* and *C. haemolyticum* because the last produce a betalike hemolysis on blood agar and do not produce the characteristic hydrogen sulfide in the butt of a TSI slant. *Listeria monocytogenes* has a characteristic tumbling motility, is usually hemolytic, ferments salicin, and hydrolyzes esculin.

■ **What characteristics do the bacteria, chlamydiae, rickettsiae, and mycoplasmas share?**

All of these are "bacterial" in characteristics. Each is characterized by the presence of both ribonucleic and deoxyribonucleic acid, binary fission as the method of reproduction, the presence of energy-yielding autonomous metabolism, antibiotic susceptibility, and the presence of ribosomes.

■ **What is BCG?**

BCG, or bacille Calmette-Guérin, is a vaccine prepared from an attenuated living avirulent strain of *Mycobacterium bovis*. The vaccine is administered intracutaneously and stimulates the production of delayed hypersensitivity and partial immunity to infection with *M. tuberculosis* and *M. bovis*. Individuals who have been vaccinated will convert and maintain a positive tuberculin reaction for many years and during this period are probably adequately protected from tuberculosis. Individuals who are tuberculin positive should not be given BCG.

This procedure has not been universally adopted. It is used in the United States in local areas in which crowding, poverty, or undernourishment prevail or in families in whom exposure to active tuberculosis infection exists. Some countries practice BCG vaccination of the total population and have been able to significantly reduce the incidence of tuberculosis.

■ **What in vivo test may be used to detect hypersensitivity to tuberculin?**

OT (old tuberculin) or PPD (purified protein derivative) are the active preparations. They may be injected intradermally (Mantoux), scratched onto the surface of the skin (Von Pirquet), applied to the skin on a patch of filter paper (Vollmer), pricked 1 to 2 mm into the skin (Heath), or introduced into the skin with a multiple puncture instrument (Tine).

■ **Which stool specimens should be processed for parasites without delay?**

All specimens should be processed without undue delay. However, it is very important to examine promptly if trophozoite movement is to be observed. A dysenteric mucus and blood-tinged stool from a patient infected with *Entamoeba histolytica* is such a specimen. Of course, it is sometimes difficult to guess the cause of dysentery or severe diarrhea. Bacillary dysentery caused by the shigellae may produce similar specimens and must be promptly processed.

■ **Many parasitic infestations can be diagnosed by the finding of cysts or trophozoites in the stool specimen. Describe the method of laboratory confirmation of trichinosis.**

Trichinosis is acquired from eating contaminated meat such as pork. The adult forms inhabit the digestive tract of man and produce larval forms that invade the tissues of the same host, without going through an intermediary host. The parasite does not occur in free form in any of its developmental phases and therefore cannot be identified from the stool specimen.

The early laboratory diagnosis is very difficult and is rarely made. During the first few days, adult worms may occasionally be observed by sedimentation of feces. From the end of the first week until the end of larval migration, larvae may be demonstrated from the blood of those heavily infected (1 to 2 larvae/ml). Biopsy of the encysted larvae may be done on the deltoid, biceps, and gastrocnemius muscles. Serologic analysis may serve as an adjunct to clinical diagnosis but is usually not specific enough to be used alone. Positive skin and precipitin tests have about the same specificity, but the skin test may be negative in very light and very heavy infestations.

■ **Differentiate *Taenia solium* from *T. saginata*.**

The larvae of *T. solium* are found in pigs (and humans), whereas the *T. saginata* is found in cattle and humans. The scolex of *T. solium* is armed with a double row of hooks, the gravid uterus has 5 to 13 branches, and the proglottids are passed in long chains. In contrast, the *T. saginata* scolex is without hooks, the gravid uterus has from 15 to 30 branches, and the proglottids are usually passed singly.

The two cannot be differentiated by the appearance of the egg.

■ **A trophozoite measuring approximately 19μ with ingested RBCs was seen in a stool specimen. What species might this represent and how would you differentiate between them?**

The size would suggest *Entamoeba coli* or a large race *E. histolytica* from a case of amebic dysentery. Although it is rare for *E. coli* to ingest RBCs, it nevertheless does happen in patients with persistent bleeding of the colon, during which time the *E. coli* become conditioned to feed on the red cells.

To eliminate this latter possibility, look for two clues: (1) Cysts are usually found even in the presence of trophozoites, unless the stool is quite liquid, or are present in an exudate. If no cysts are found, ask for repeat specimens until a cyst-bearing stool is obtained. (2) Look at a fresh stool for the presence of progressive crawling trophozoite motility. The nucleus of *E. coli* trophozoites is visible, but a nucleus is not usually seen in trophozoites of *E. histolytica*. If both of these fail, make stained smears for differentiation of the ameba or induce constipation to obtain stools with cysts.

■ **A pear-shaped (anteroposterior view) and a spoon-shaped (lateral view) trophozoite measuring about 12μ to 15μ in length with a slow tumbling or fallen-leaf motion was seen in a duodenal aspirate. Name the probable organism and state the clinical significance.**

Giardia lamblia is probably present. Giardiasis is an infestation of the intestinal tract of man occurring primarily in the duodenum and jejunum. Chronic diarrhea is the most common symptom in adults, occasionally coexisting with steatorrhea and malabsorption. Children are more susceptible to giardiasis than adults.

Epigastric pain, vague abdominal discomfort, loss of appetite, fever, weight loss, and symptoms referable to the liver and gallbladder, e.g., jaundice, may be present. However, many people harbor the parasite in an essentially commensal relationship without symptoms.

■ **A patient who had recently returned from a malarial zone was found to have fever every fourth day. On examination of the blood smear a mature schizont was seen to contain 6 merozoites. What malarial parasite might this represent and how would you confirm this?**

This suggests *Plasmodium malariae* infection, the cause of quartan malaria. One should also look for other parasites of different maturation. *P. malariae* rarely has more than one parasite per red cell and has coarse pigment granules in the growing trophozoite. The growing schizonts are compact, oval or round, with 2 to 6 chromatin granules and coarse granules or clumps of pigment. The mature schizont has 6 to 12 merozoites, forming a single ring or cluster resembling a rosette or a daisy, and has the pigment located as a central mass.

■ **What is the exoerythrocytic cycle of malarial parasites?**

This is a schizogonic stage of development of the malarial parasite that takes place in the reticuloendothelial system and other tissues and is characterized by a lack of malarial pigment. It is thought to develop as certain merozoites of the erythrocytic cycle enter tissue cells or as a result of tissue cell invasion by the macromerozoites that were produced earlier during the preerythrocytic stages.

■ *Trypanosoma gambiense* and *T. rhodensiense* cause African sleeping sickness. How could infection with either of these parasites be confirmed in the laboratory?

The trypanosomes may be demonstrated from lymph node aspirates, blood, or cerebrospinal fluid. In early disease, the enlarged lymph node is the best site from which to obtain material; later the organisms may be readily recovered from blood and occasionally from CSF. Direct examination is the best method of demonstrating the parasites, although culture is sometimes beneficial.

In the cover-slipped fresh wet blood mount, movement of the parasite causes characteristic movement of the blood cells. If blood smears are prepared, they should be stained in the same manner as for malarial parasites. Blood concentration employing 2% citrate as an anticoagulant and 2% acetic acid as a lysing solution followed by centrifugation has permitted visualization of parasites in light infections. Inoculation of 2 to 10 ml of blood into guinea pigs, mice, or rats may produce a positive infection in a week or so.

■ What parasite causes visceral leishmaniasis and what is its morphologic form?

Leishmania donovani appears in man only in the leishmanial form. It is an intracellular, oval, and nonflagellated body found especially in the cells of the reticuloendothelial system but occasionally in small numbers in the blood. When stained with Giemsa or Wright's stain, a large red nucleus and a purple rod-shaped parabasal body are readily seen. Single macrophages may be heavily parasitized with these bodies.

■ What are viruses?

Viruses, or virions, are small infectious agents that are potentially pathogenic in the susceptible host. They contain either deoxyribonucleic acid or ribonucleic acid, but not both, which is situated in a core covered by a protein sheath, or capsid. The capsid is composed of protein subunits that are packed very closely together in either cubical or helical symmetrical patterns. The host cell replicates more of these infectious units from the viral genetic material. Viruses are insensitive to the effects of antibiotics, which are effective against bacteria.

■ What is the basis of classification of viruses?

Viruses may be classified in many ways. Clinicians classify them according to the clinical disease associated with them. Virologists classify them according to their nucleic acid content, size, morphology, ether sensitivity, heat lability, and pH lability.

■ **Define tropism as it relates to "target organs."**

An early classification based on the affinity for and localization of a virus in specific tissues (e.g., skin by dermotropic, paralysis by neurotropic, pneumonia by pneumotropic, and enteritis by enterotropic virus) was thought to be highly specifiic. Although tropisms do exist because of specific receptors localized in the tissues, these characteristics are not stable enough for purposes of classification. Many viruses have no specific tissue affinities. The Coxsackie B virus, for example, can infect such diverse tissues as muscle, brain, meninges, subcutaneous fat, pancreas, heart, and pericardium. Thus, tropism offers the least reliable of all factors that can be used in the classification of viruses.

■ **What is the significance of antibodies to the Epstein-Barr virus?**

This herpeslike virus was originally observed in cell cultures from the highly malignant Burkitt's lymphoma common in central and east African children. This virus has been implicated in infectious mononucleosis; all patients with the infectious mononucleosis syndrome who are infected with this virus as well as all patients with Burkitt's lymphoma have demonstrable antibodies to this agent. This antibody is quite distinct from the heterophile antibody.

■ **What are blastospores and what is the method of reproduction in them?**

Blastospores are round to pyriform asexual reproductive units of yeast and yeastlike organisms. Most reproduce by single budding, but *Paracoccidioides braziliensis* characteristically has multiple budding. Daughter buds are usually joined to the parent blastospore by a narrow point of attachment. However, daughter blastospores of *Blastomyces dermatitidis* are attached by a broad base and have a wide pore between them.

■ **What are arthrospores and which fungi possess them?**

Arthrospores are one of three types of thallospores, which are asexual reproductive spores formed from the thallus or mycelium. The arthrospore is formed by segmentation of the hyphae to form rectangular thick-walled cells. *Geotrichum, Oidium* or *Oospora,* and *Coccidioides* reproduce in this manner in culture. In addition, the dermatophytes exhibit this type of sporulation in tissue.

■ **What is a germ tube and how is the phenomenon of germ tube formation used in the clinical laboratory?**

The germ tube is a short filament arising from a blastospore of *Candida*. If the test is carried out in egg albumin, human serum, or some other similar medium at 37° C and is read within 2 hours, it is reported to be quite specific for *Candida albicans*. It is a useful tool for presumptive identification of colonies of *C. albicans* from clinical material. *C. stellatoidea* may also have a positive germ tube in 2 hours at 37° C.

■ **Which fungi may appear as "yeast" forms in human tissue?**

Candida, Cryptococcus, Torulopsis, Geotrichum, Sporothrix (Sporotrichum), Blastomyces, Paracoccidioides, Coccidioides, Histoplasma, and *Loboa* appear as "yeast" forms.

■ **What is the usefulness and limitation of a KOH mount of skin scrapings?**

It is useful to digest the keratinized cells and permit the fungal elements to be visualized. One can differentiate between cutaneous dermatophyte infections and those caused by *Candida*. However, all dermatophytes of the genera *Trichophyton, Microsporum,* and *Epidermophyton* produce arthrospores that are identical to one another.

■ **Of what use is Wood's light?**

Wood's light is an ultraviolet light with an emission at 3,650 Å. A shaft of hair infected with *Trichophyton schoenleini* will fluoresce a bluish white, and one infected with *Microsporum* species, except *M. gypseum,* will fluoresce a greenish yellow when illuminated with this light in a darkened room. This enables the selection of parasitized hair for examination and culture. A 100-watt Blak-Ray lamp or one of comparable intensity is recommended.

■ **Why is an India ink preparation performed and what are the benefits and limitations of the procedure?**

An India ink preparation is a negative capsule stain used to demonstrate encapsulated blastospores of *Cryptococcus neoformans* in cerebrospinal fluid of patients with *C. neoformans* meningitis. A positive finding of fully encapsulated blastospores that are budding is diagnostic. However, only about 50% of patients with *C. neoformans* meningitis have a positive India ink preparation. For this reason, all suspect spinal fluids must be cultured on Sabouraud's or similar media for this organism. One must exercise caution in interpreting the smear inasmuch as a lymphocyte may simulate a *C. neoformans* blastospore with a small capsule.

■ **Identify** *Candida albicans.*

Candida albicans is a yeastlike fungus that is worldwide in distribution. In humans it is found readily as part of skin, vaginal, oral, and gut normal flora. Under proper circumstances the organism can cause local infections on the skin and mucous membranes or become systemic and cause lesions in the lung or kidneys or metastatic lesions throughout the body. It is characterized by its ability to form germ tubes in human serum in 2 hours at 37° C, to consistently ferment glucose and maltose, and to assimilate glucose, maltose, sucrose, galactose, xylose, and trehalose.

■ **How is candidemia best detected?**

Candidemia may be either transient or associated with *Candida* sepsis. In either instance, the most sensitive and rapid method for isolation is to collect blood with Liquoid (SPS, or sodium polyanethol sulfonate), lyse with Triton X-100 (alkyl phenoxy polyethoxy ethanol) and sodium carbonate, and filter onto a membrane with 0.45μ porosity. The filter should be washed with sterile saline solution and aseptically placed onto the agar surface of some suitable agar in a Petri dish. Growth will almost always appear within 24 hours.

■ **What is thrush?**

Thrush is oral candidiasis caused by *Candida albicans* and characterized by discrete or confluent patches of a cream-white to gray pseudomembrane on the tongue, soft palate, or buccal mucosa. It is found more frequently in the newborn, who is probably contaminated in the birth canal, and in those who are aged, have a debilitating disease, are on broad-spectrum antibiotics, or are diabetic.

■ **What parasite does the tissue form of** *Histoplasma capsulatum* **resemble and how can it be differentiated?**

The intracellular forms of *H. capsulatum* are small spherical or ovoid bodies in histiocytes that measure 1μ to 5μ in diameter and under low magnification on H&E stain resemble *Leishmania*. If the material is well fixed and viewed under high-power magnification, the kinetoplast of the *Leishmania* should be visible. Any of the special fungus stains, such as Gridley, periodic acid–Schiff, or Gomori methenamine silver, will stain the *Histoplasma* fungus but will not stain the *Leishmania* parasites.

■ **What fungi are characterized by producing one morphologic form in** tissue and a very dissimilar form on culture and are thus designated as diphasic?

Blastomyces dermatitidis, Coccidioides immitis, Histoplasma capsulatum, Sporothrix (Sporotrichum) schenckii, and *Paracoccidioides braziliensis* are diphasic fungi.

■ **Describe the appearance of** *Coccidioides immitis* **in tissue.**

The majority of organisms in tissue resemble the nonbudding forms of *Blastomyces dermatitidis* or *Paracoccidioides braziliensis.* They have thick double-contoured walls and may vary from 2μ to 200μ in diameter. The material stains in an irregular fashion in the young developing spherule, but as it becomes a more mature spherule it is found to contain many endospores or sporangiospores. The histologic picture will vary from an early pyogenic reaction similar to the response to bacteria to a granulomatous response of histiocytic exudate and giant cells resulting from reaction to the sporangium.

■ **What similarities exist in the tissue response among** *Mycobacterium tuberculosis* **and the various systemic fungi?**

A very important reaction in tuberculosis is related to cell-mediated hypersensitivity. The giant cells, tubercle formation, and other granulomatous reactions are reactions to the tuberculoprotein. In like manner, granulomatous reactions or the hypersensitivity components are frequently the most prominent aspect of systemic fungus infections.

■ **What are antibodies?**

Antibodies are globulin protein molecules (immunoglobulins) formed in a susceptible host as a result of stimulation by an antigen (immunogen). They characteristically react specifically with the related antigen in some demonstrable manner.

■ **What is the generally accepted theory of antibody formation?**

The selective theory, advanced by Sir McFarland Burnet, holds that the information required for the synthesis of different antibodies already resides in the genetic apparatus before exposure to the antigen or immunogen. When contact is made between the immunogen and the proper cell, the gene that is responsible for coding a specific antibody protein is selected and "turned on." Through transcription and translation of the appropriate messenger RNA, specific peptide (immunoglobulin) chains, along with their corresponding individual primary amino acid sequences, are synthesized. As a result of this sequence, the chains fold spontaneously into a preferred globular configuration that has the specific antigen or immunogen combining sites.

■ **What is the difference between "affinity" and "avidity" as applied to antigen-antibody reactions?**

The term "affinity" is used to describe the equilibrium for the reaction between an antigen binding site on the antibody and the determinant on the immunogen (e.g., monovalent hapten), whereas the term "avidity" is applied to the reaction between whole molecules of antigen and antibody when the valency of the reactants becomes involved.

■ **What is an anamnestic response?**

This secondary, or memory, response is observed on second exposure to an antigen. Antibodies or immunocompetent cells are produced more rapidly, and the latent period is shortened or nonexistent. Antibody levels are higher and persist longer than in the primary response. IgG is the principal antibody produced.

■ **What bioactive products are produced by the complement sequence?**

C1,4 results in the neutralization of herpes simplex viruses that have been sensitized by IgM antibody.

C1,4,2 is thought to produce a kininlike material that will contract smooth muscle and cause increased vascular permeability. This kininlike material is resistant to the antihistamine drugs.

C3b, attached to a red cell, may lead to rapid cell destruction, recognized as autoimmune hemolytic disorder. On the surface of red cells, platelets, or leukocytes, C3b will bring out immune adherence. This is a phenomenon in which each cell will cause attachment or adherence to normal RBCs with resulting agglutination in vitro.

C3a biotoxic activities include anaphylatoxin, which causes contraction of smooth muscle, release of histamine from mast cells, and increased vascular permeability, and a second action of induction of leukocyte chemotaxis or the attraction of neutrophilic granulocytes in a unidirectional manner.

C5a, in a manner analogous to C3a, has anaphylatoxic and chemotactic properties for granulocytes. It is thought that C5b is important in some phagocytic systems.

C5, 6, 7, or activated trimolecular complex, has chemotactic activity for neutrophils.

It is known that if C8 and C9 react with the earlier portion of the

complement sequence in proximity to a cell surface, a cytotoxic alteration of the membrane occurs, resulting in the loss of the functional integrity of the cells and the loss of cellular constituents. Such cells are
irreversibly damaged.

■ **What are complement fixation tests?**

Complement fixation tests, complement-dependent lytic reactions,
are in vitro manifestations of antigen-antibody interaction. These reactions form the basis for laboratory tests used in the detection and identification of antigens and antibodies involved in disease processes.

■ **Where does complement react with the immunoglobulin molecule?**

Complement reacts with the Fc portion of the antibody molecule.
Different immunoglobulin classes have different Fc structures, and
not all will bind complement. This characteristic is shared only by
IgM and IgG. There are even differences among the various subclasses of IgG: IgG_1 and IgG_3 fix complement well, IgG_2 less so, and IgG_4
poorly if at all. The Clq molecule, which is linked in a trimolecular
complex to Clr and Cls, is polyvalent and needs to combine with at
least two Fc sites for activation. This presents no problem with the
pentavalent IgM molecule, because several Fc regions are readily
available within one molecule. However, IgG can fix complement
only when two or more molecules are bound to adjacent sites on the
antigen.

■ **What is the significance of IgM in the infectious process?**

IgM is the immunoglobulin class that has the greatest antibacterial
activity. IgM is formed early in the immune response and serves as an
opsonin, promoting phagocytosis. It immobilizes bacteria by agglutination and causes lysis by efficient activation of complement.

■ **What are reagins?**

Reagins are IgE antibodies that mediate "allergic" or "atopic"
states. They compose a very small part (0.002%) of the total serum
immunoglobulin. There is a cytophilic affinity of the Fc portion of IgE
(ε-chain) and the membrane of mast cells, neutrophils, and basophils.
IgE can sensitize these cells to allergens and, on subsequent contact
with the allergen, will immediately undergo degranulation with the
release of vasoactive substances such as histamine and histaminelike
substances.

■ **What is transfer factor?**

Transfer factor is a dialyzable polypeptide extracted from human
lymphocytes and is capable of transferring cell-mediated immunity to

a number of antigens, including tuberculin and diphtheria toxoid. Its precise mode of action is unknown.

■ **What is lymphotoxin (LT)?**

Lymphotoxin is a heat-stable substance with a molecular weight of about 80,000 to 150,000 that has been liberated from specifically sensitized lymphocytes as well as from lymphocytes stimulated by nonspecific stimulators, such as phytohemagglutinin (PHA). This substance seemingly inhibits the capacity of cells to undergo division and is associated with target cell injury.

■ **How is it thought that the immune response system plays a role in the pathogenesis of poststreptococcal glomerulonephritis?**

Following an upper respiratory tract infection with certain types of Group A *Streptococcus pyogenes*, antistreptococcal antibodies are formed. These antibodies complex with circulating streptococcal antigens and are filtered out by the renal glomeruli and deposited in the Bowman's space aspect of the capillary basement membrane. Subsequent binding of complement initiates acute inflammation of the glomeruli with increased glomerular permeability, leading to the leakage of proteins and cells into the urine.

Immunofluorescent procedures demonstrate "lumpy-bumpy" deposits of IgG and complement on the outside of the glomerular basement membrane.

■ **What two dissimilar populations of small lymphocytes are present and to what phase of the immune response are they related?**

T-lymphocytes are processed by or are in some way dependent on the thymus. These small lymphocytes are responsible for cell-mediated hypersensitivity, e.g., tuberculin hypersensitivity.

B-lymphocytes are bursa dependent, at least as demonstrated in the chicken, and are concerned with the synthesis of circulating antibody. In humans and other mammals, no specific anatomic structure, such as the bursa of Fabricius, has been found. However, gut-associated lymphoid tissue such as the tonsil, Peyer's patches, and appendix are thought to serve this purpose.

■ **Can a primary T-cell deficiency predispose an individual to bacterial infection?**

We are aware that the T-cell small lymphocytes are related to cell-mediated hypersensitivity and the ability to handle viral infections. However, the ability to handle bacteria that have a hypersensitivity component depends on the presence of a functional T-cell system.

Thus, even the administration of the attenuated BCG or attenuated *Mycobacterium bovis* vaccine can be devastating to a child with primary T-cell deficiency.

■ **How would a primary B-cell deficiency manifest itself in a child?**

The child would be expected to have normal cell-mediated immune responses and would have the ability to readily handle viral infections such as measles and smallpox.

However, inasmuch as the humoral response would be depressed, the production of specific immunoglobulins would be grossly depressed, and the child would be subject to repeated infection with pyogenic bacteria, such as *Staphylococcus aureus, Streptococcus pyogenes, S. pneumoniae, Neisseria meningitidis,* and *Haemophilus influenzae.* In addition, *Candida albicans,* a fungus, and *Pneumocystis carinii,* a protozoan, could cause severe infections. Histologically, there would be few lymphoid follicles or plasma cells present in lymph node biopsies.

■ **Can an antibody molecule react with the Fab and Fc portions at the same time?**

Yes. In the classic reaction, the Fab portion of the immunoglobulin combines with the immunogen or homologous antigen. However, the antibody to the class of immunoglobulin or its heavy chain could react with the Fc portion. Thus, we would react antigen versus antibody in a classic agar gel precipitation reaction and then react a radioactive-tagged antibody to the different heavy chains to discover the class of antibody of immunoglobulin that was entering into the reaction.

■ **How do the various serologic tests compare in sensitivity when measuring antibody nitrogen of high-avidity antibody?**

The precipitin and immunoelectrophoresis tests are the least sensitive, requiring 3 to 20 mg Ab N/ml/test. Double diffusion in agar gel is slightly more sensitive, requiring 0.2 to 1.0 mg Ab N/ml/test. At the other end of the spectrum are the virus neutralization and bactericidal tests, which require 1×10^{-4} to 1×10^{-5} mg Ab N, and laser nephelometry, which requires only 1×10^{-9} mg Ab/ml. The radioimmunoassay and antigen-combining globulin technique (Farr) requires 1×10^{-3} to 1×10^{-4} mg.

The intermediate tests are complement fixation, 0.01 to 0.1; radial immunodiffusion, 0.008 to 0.025; bacterial agglutination, 0.01; hemolysis, 0.001 to 0.03; passive hemagglutination, 0.005; and antitoxin neutralization, 0.003 mg Ab N/ml/test.

The in vivo passive cutaneous anaphylaxis test requires 0.003 mg

Ab N. Accordingly, one must select the test with the proper sensitivity if one wishes to perform serologic quantitation of antibody.

■ **What is the rheumatoid factor and what is its clinical significance?**

The rheumatoid factor is a macroglobulin or immunoglobulin belonging to the IgM class that is found primarily in the alpha globulin, although to some extent it may be found in the beta fraction of serum. It may be found in the serum of rheumatoid arthritis and SLE patients even though they may lack the clinical manifestations of the disease. Trauma, fatigue, and emotional factors have also been incriminated as possible etiologic or precipitating factors. The factor agglutinates a variety of suspended particles, including hemolytic streptococci, sheep RBCs sensitized with antisheep erythrocyte rabbit serum, latex, and bentonite suspensions.

Significant titers for rheumatoid arthritis vary with the test procedure. For the sheep cell agglutinin it is 232; bentonite, 32; and latex, 20. The hemagglutinin reaction with sensitized sheep erythrocytes, although positive in up to 90% of cases of rheumatoid arthritis, is also positive in 15% to 25% of SLE cases, in an occasional case of sarcoidosis, syphilis, and scleroderma, and in 1% to 4% of normal human sera.

■ **How does cross-reactivity influence the interpretation of immunodiagnostic tests for unknown fevers?**

The febrile agglutination tests are used to detect antibodies to various bacteria, e.g., *Salmonella, Brucella, Francisella tularensis,* and *Rickettsia.* Inasmuch as many of the *Salmonella* antigens are shared with various members of the genus and family, there will be cross-agglutination whenever this occurs. However, if a battery of antigens is used, the agglutination will occur more quickly and will be stronger with the homologous antigen than with the minor or cross-reacting one.

Of course, cross-reaction is the basis of the detection of *Rickettsia* antibodies with suspensions of various *Proteus* strains in the Weil-Felix reaction. In addition, a good history is important to evaluate the agglutination reactions with *Brucella* and *Francisella tularensis* antigens.

■ **Define and discuss the clinical significance of the C-reactive protein.**

The C-reactive protein is an abnormal protein that appears in the blood of patients with acute inflammatory reactions but is absent in healthy individuals. It is an alpha globulin whose production is stimulated by various bacterial infections, pyrogenic agents, or products of injured tissue. It is predictably present in rheumatic activity and serves as a sensitive and reliable indicator of inflammatory activity. Conversely, the disappearance of the C-reactive protein reflects effective treatment or spontaneous remission.

■ **What is the Weil-Felix test?**

The Weil-Felix test is an agglutination procedure used to detect antibodies to various rickettsiae belonging to the genus *Rickettsia* but not the genus *Coxiella*. The antigen used in this test is one of several strains of *Proteus* designated OX-19, OX-2, and OX-K. Although low titers of agglutinins may be found in an infection with *Proteus*, titers of several hundred are found with the typhus fevers and Rocky Mountain spotted fever.

■ **What is the significance of cold agglutinins or cold-reacting antibodies?**

Antibodies for human type O erythrocytes active at 0° to 10° C may be found in a variety of acute infections, such as *Mycoplasma pneumoniae*, infectious mononucleosis, trypanosomiasis, and congenital cytomegalovirus infection. The common use of this test is in the patient with primary atypical pneumonia (PAP) caused by *M. pneumoniae*. Although cold agglutinins appear in only about 50% of the mild cases of infectious mononucleosis, they are present in greater percentage and are found in higher titer in severe cases.

■ **What are Forssman antibodies?**

Forssman antibodies belong to the class of heterophile antibodies. Immunization of rabbits with guinea pig tissues stimulates the production of antibodies that agglutinate sheep RBCs. These non–species-specific antibodies are Forssman antibodies.

■ **What relationship do the heterophile antibodies have to infectious mononucleosis?**

Antisheep or heterophile agglutinins may be found in low titer in normal individuals. During infectious mononucleosis, the heterophile antibody titer may increase to 224 or greater. This, coupled with characteristic clinical symptoms, is presumptive evidence of this disease.

Heterophile antibodies may be observed in serum sickness. To differentiate among these three heterophile antibodies, the serum should be adsorbed with guinea pig extract to remove the agglutinins of serum sickness or the naturally occurring heterophile antibody. The heterophile antibody of infectious mononucleosis is not removed by guinea pig adsorption but is removed by ox cell adsorption.

■ **What serologic tests can be used to evaluate the patient for recent streptococcal infection?**

Antistreptolysin O, antihyaluronidase, and antideoxyribonuclease tests are the tests of choice. Generally, although antistreptolysin O is the most sensitive test in pharyngeal infections, antideoxyribonuclease is the most sensitive in skin infections.

■ **How does immunization affect the typhoid O and H antibodies in the Widal test?**

Immunization causes an increase in the H agglutinins. However, active infection causes an early increase in O agglutinins followed by an increase in H agglutinins, which persist longer. The presence of H agglutinins only would suggest a previous infection or immunization, whereas positive reactions involving the O antigens would be more suggestive of an active infection.

■ **Discuss the laboratory aids available to assist in the diagnosis of brucellosis.**

A positive culture is the most reliable indicator of brucellosis. The next most reliable test is the agglutinin test. Titers of 320 or greater are usually found in the active case. A fourfold increase in titer is necessary for a serologic diagnosis. However, even some patients with a positive blood culture have low titers of antibodies or occasionally are negative altogether. The presence of incomplete and blocking antibodies must be considered. The prozone phenomenon has been demonstrated up to titers of 400, but this can be minimized by use of a 5% NaCl solution as the diluent. The incomplete antibodies can be detected with Coombs' serum.

■ **What is the principle of the VDRL slide test for syphilis?**

The VDRL antigen is composed of purified cardiolipin and lecithin from beef heart, with cholesterol added to increase the antigen's effective reacting surface. Reagin from syphilis, or any other disease that produces reagin, causes dispersion of the cardiolipin-lecithin antigen that is observed as a visible flocculation.

■ **What is the usefulness of the FTA-ABS test in evaluating the questionable syphilitic patient?**

The FTA-ABS test is an indirect fluorescent antibody test devised to detect antibodies in the patient's serum that are specific for the spirochete *Treponema pallidum*. In the procedure, the nonspecific reacting substances in the serum are removed by a sorbent prepared from a sonication of the nonpathogenic Reiter treponeme. Thus, antibodies "specific" for the *T. pallidum* remain in the serum. Although a rare serum will still exhibit fluorescence in the absence of syphilis, the test remains one of the most reliable and easily performed of current syphilis serologic procedures.

The FTA-ABS test becomes reactive about as quickly as the reagin tests (VDRL, RPR, etc.) in primary syphilis—3 to 4 weeks—but remains reactive even after effective therapy. Thus, the FTA-ABS test is the one to be used for confirmation of syphilis or to rule out syphilis when the commonly used screening tests detect nonsyphilitic reagin.

■ **When would a spinal fluid VDRL examination be indicated?**

When there is a suspicion of neurosyphilis. False-positive reactions in the CSF are very rare. The presence of reagin in the CSF is the only finding that is highly indicative and a reliable indicator of present or past neurosyphilis. A diagnosis of latent syphilis can be confirmed only if asymptomatic neurosyphilis is ruled out by a negative reagin test of the CSF.

■ **How does the RPR card test compare with other serologic tests for syphilis?**

The RPR, or rapid plasma reagin, card test has the same significance as any other reagin test when reactive or nonreactive. Its sensitivity and specificity are comparable to those of the VDRL. However, the antigen in the RPR test is much more stable than the VDRL, and RPR is the preferred test when experts trained in the preparation of the VDRL antigen of standard reactivity are not available. This includes developing countries, field laboratories, small laboratories that perform only occasional serologic tests for syphilis, and indeed even many of the serologic units in some larger hospitals.

■ **Describe the principle of the hemagglutination-inhibition test and its diagnostic importance.**

Certain viruses have the ability to agglutinate erythrocytes from various species. This activity can be inhibited by specific antibody. Thus, antibodies in serum against viruses such as influenza, measles, and rubella can be detected by serum's ability to inhibit the viral hemagglutinating activity.

■ **What is counterimmunoelectrophoresis? What is its most common laboratory application?**

Counterimmunoelectrophoresis is a modification of immunoelectrophoresis in which antigen and antibody are driven toward each other by an electrical field. This speeds the reaction and increases its sensitivity. This procedure is most commonly used to detect hepatitis-associated antigen (HAA).

■ **Describe the principle of radial immunodiffusion. For what is this technique used?**

Specific antisera are incorporated into an agar gel for unknown sera and known standards. A known amount of serum is placed in the wells, and plates are incubated in a moist chamber at room temperature. The proteins diffuse from the wells into the gel. The specific antigen combines with the antibody in the gel, forming a circular precipitation line. The diameter of this circle is proportional to the concentration of antigen in the serum.

This procedure may be used to quantitate serum components such as immunoglobulins, transferrin, complement C3, and $alpha_1$-antitrypsin.

■ **What abnormality in serum immunoglobulins is often associated with helminth infection?**

Increased levels of IgE are commonly observed in patients with parasitic diseases. Other allergic manifestations, such as urticaria, asthma, and rashes, also characterize these diseases. It is thought that IgE may function as a local defense against parasitic disease.

■ **Discuss the significance of rubella antibody titers.**

Rubella is a generally benign viral infection unless acquired during the first trimester of intrauterine life. In utero infection is associated with a very high incidence of severe fetal abnormalities, and for this reason the status of the mother is important. Rubella antibody titers are generally determined by the hemagglutination inhibition technique. This technique has a high correlation with neutralization antibody titers, which technically are more difficult to determine. A titer of 1:20 is generally considered protective; a titer of 1:10 is borderline; and a titer lower than 1:10 indicates susceptibility to rubella.

■ **Discuss the significance of hepatitis B surface antigen (HB$_s$Ag).**

Hepatitis B surface antigen, which was previously called Australia antigen or hepatitis-associated antigen, is an antigen of the capsid of the hepatitis B virus. It is important for a number of reasons. In people with symptoms of acute viral hepatitis who are known to have been HB$_s$Ag negative in the past, a positive test establishes the diagnosis of acute type B viral hepatitis. The persistence of the surface antigen in people with acute type B viral hepatitis suggests that the disease may be progressing to chronic active hepatitis. Screening for HB$_s$Ag is also important in blood donors, because a significant number of people with HB$_s$Ag have complete infectious viruses in their serum and are capable of transmitting type B hepatitis in transfused blood.

■ **What is a biologic false-positive VDRL test and what is its significance?**

The VDRL test for syphilis is a nonspecific test, and a number of other conditions may cause the reaction to be positive. Those positive reactions not caused by syphilis or technical problems are called biologic false-positives. Biologic false-positives usually have titers of less than 1:8. These reactions are divided into acute and chronic false-positives. The acute reaction lasts less than 6 months. It is associated with a number of infectious diseases, including pneumonia, tuberculosis, endocarditis, chickenpox, and infectious mononucleosis. The chronic form of biologic false-positive VDRL is associated with the so-called autoimmune diseases, especially SLE. In addition, biologic false-positives are more common in elderly patients. It is estimated that as many as 10% of people age 80 or more have a false-positive VDRL reaction.

■ **What are antinuclear antibodies and what is their significance?**

Demonstration of antinuclear antibodies followed as a natural outgrowth the demonstration of the LE cell phenomenon in SLE. Indeed, these antibodies in serum lead to the production of the LE cell. Thus, antinuclear antibodies are antibodies to components of the cell's nucleus. They are present in a large variety of so-called collagen vascular diseases and are not specific for SLE.

■ **What is the significance of mitochondrial antibodies?**

Mitochondrial antibodies are useful in the differential diagnosis of patients with chronic liver diseases. They are present in high titer in more than 90% of cases of primary biliary cirrhosis. They are absent in cases of extrahepatic biliary obstruction.

CHAPTER 7

Instrumentation and quality control

John D. Reeves

■ **Distinguish between photometer, colorimeter, and spectrophotometer.**

The photometer is any instrument that measures the intensity of a beam of light. In the clinical laboratory, the term colorimeter specifically refers to the instrument used to measure the intensity of colored light. It is understood that the color (range of wavelengths) used is selected by some sort of filter, thus the alternate designation of filter photometer. A spectrophotometer also measures light intensity; but, with the addition of a device to disperse the source light into a continuous spectrum, it permits the selection of any desired wavelength in the available range and provides improved control over the range of adjacent wavelengths included in the beam produced.

■ **What is monochromatic light and what devices can be used to produce it?**

Monochromatic light literally means "light of one color." In spectrophotometry, we would like to consider true monochromatic light to be defined as light radiation of a single wavelength, although what a monochromator provides in practice is always a range of wavelengths on both sides of the desired one. The average spectral width of this range expressed in units of wavelength is the band pass; this is the characteristic that distinguishes different monochromator systems.

The major monochromating devices are the following.

1. The colored filter, usually glass, absorbs some portions of the electromagnetic spectrum and transmits others. Light energy is absorbed by dye compounds in the glass and is ultimately dissipated as heat. The band pass is quite wide, perhaps 35 to 50 nm or more.

2. The interference filter utilizes the wave character of light to enhance the intensity of the desired wavelength by constructive interference and eliminates other wavelengths by destructive interference and reflection. The band pass can be limited to 10 to 20 nm with these filters.

3. A prism disperses white light into a continuous spectrum of colors based on small differences in refractive index for different wavelengths of light, red light having a lower refractive index than the shorter violet light. Any band of wavelengths can be isolated by projecting this spectrum onto the exit slit. The band pass can be limited to a few nanometers, although this becomes increasingly difficult toward the long wave regions, where the nonlinear dispersion of the prism results in a crowded spectrum.

4. The most common dispersing device used today, particularly in the lower cost spectrophotometers for clinical laboratory applications, is the diffraction grating. It is generally manufactured as a replica grating. Gratings may be of either the transmission or reflectance type, although both are basically pieces of optical glass with very closely spaced precision parallel grooves (approximately 15,000 per inch). The spectrum is produced by interference resulting from small path differences between light waves as they are scattered by the narrow grooves. The grating has two advantages over the prism as a dispersing devise: (1) it produces a linear spectrum, and therefore, maintaining a constant band pass is simple; and (2) it can be used in the regions of the spectrum where light energy is absorbed by glass prisms (ultraviolet and infrared).

■ **Define nominal wavelength and band pass width.**

The nominal wavelength is the one that is read off the selection dial of the spectrophotometer and is located in the center of the spectral segment of wavelengths that actually pass through the exit slit to form the final beam of monochromatic light. In the spectrophotometer, the band pass depends on the design of the monochromator but is essentially equivalent to the spectral width (in nanometers) of the exit slit. Note that nonlinear dispersion of a prism will result in a variable spectral width when a fixed-width exit slit is used. For a filter, the true definition of band pass is more explanatory: the range of wavelengths between the two points where transmission intensity is one-half that of the transmission peak (which occurs at the nominal wavelength).

■ **Describe four different types of photodetectors.**

1. The photovoltaic cell, formerly referred to as a barrier layer cell, is commonly constructed of a plate of metal (e.g., iron) covered with a thin layer of a photosensitive semiconductor material (e.g., selenium). Light radiation forces electrons out of the crystal structure of the semiconductor, creating a population of free electrons and a population of positively charged "holes" (vacancies left by escaped electrons). This difference in charge distribution on the two surfaces of the cell results in a measurable voltage that is directly proportional to the light intensity. The photovoltaic cell remains unique among photodetectors because it can generate its own power. The output of the cell can be measured directly with a galvanometer (microammeter) without additional circuitry. The spectral sensitivity of this device resembles that of the human eye (400 to 800nm) and is most sensitive to light of about 550 nm.

2. The photoemissive tube consists of two electrodes sealed in an evacuated glass envelope. The cathode is coated with a photosensitive mixture that emits electrons when struck by light radiation. The anode is maintained at a high positive potential and attracts the released electrons, resulting in a flow of photocurrent through the tube. The spectral sensitivity of a phototube is determined by the composition of the cathode coating. Many types are available between about 200 and 1,000 nm.

3. The photomultiplier tube uses the same principle as the photoemissive tube but uses a series of additional electrodes (dynodes) to internally amplify the photosignal before it leaves the tube. The original electrons from the photocathode are accelerated through a series of dynodes, each maintained at a higher positive potential than the last and each coated with a material that will easily release electrons. The photocurrent increases geometrically through the cascade, resulting in a high output signal for a very low-level original input of radiant energy.

4. Junction photodiodes and phototransistors are light-sensitive semiconductor devices coming into use in some clinical laboratory equipment. These are both generally operated as photoconductive-type devices. They increase their ability to conduct reverse current when light is focused on the semiconductor junction (the base of the transistor). These both require an external power source and exhibit dark current like photo-

tubes. The spectral sensitivity ranges from about 400 to 1,000 nm, with peak sensitivity around 800 nm.

■ **List several different types of readout devices used in laboratory instruments.**

Some readout devices are: (1) meter, (2) mechanical digital counter, (3) digital vacuum tubes, (4) LED (light-emitting diodes), (5) CRT (cathode-ray tubes), (6) line printers, (7) strip chart recorders, and (8) liquid crystal digital readout.

■ **What is the significance of the combined laws referred to as Beer's law?**

Beer's law is fundamental to quantitative absorption photometry. It relates the reduction of radiant power (intensity) of a beam of monochromatic light to the concentration of a sample solute of interest. The law is variously stated as:

$$\left\{ \log \frac{I_0}{I} \text{ or } \log \frac{1}{T} \text{ or } 2\text{-}\log \%T \text{ or } A \right\} = abc$$

where

I_0 = Intensity of light incident on sample
I = Intensity of light transmitted through sample
T = Transmittance (a defined term equal to $\frac{I}{I_0}$)
$\%T$ = $T \times 100$
A = Absorbance (a defined term equal to $\log \frac{1}{T}$)

a = Absorptivity (a constant, characteristic of absorbing specie)
b = Thickness of absorbing solution (optical light path)
c = Concentration of absorbing specie in light path

Note that absorbance has been defined so as to make things easier to work with, since it is a linear function with respect to concentration. Calibration curves with concentration plotted against absorbance produce a straight line on graph paper with linear coordinates. The graphic plotting of T or %T versus concentration produces an exponential curve on linear coordinates, although a straight line can be obtained by plotting log %T versus concentration (semilog chart paper simplifies handling of the log values). The practical application of Beer's law includes some very important assumptions about the nature of the absorbing specie and the conditions under which the analysis is made. These can be directly evaluated by experimentally determining the relationship between absorbance and concentration for the system of interest. One of the most important assumptions is that one is using a truly monochromatic light source. As a wider band pass is employed, deviations from the predicted linear relationship become more apparent. However, useful quantitative results may still be obtained with the careful use of a standard curve and adequate quality control.

■ **Describe the rationale for the selection of the best wavelength for quantitative determinations by absorption spectrophotometry.**

The spectral absorption curve for the compound of interest will indicate the regions of the spectrum where absorbance is maximal as well as minimal. The wavelengths of these absorption peaks are characteristic of the structure of the compound, and in the visible and ultraviolet regions they are related to the energy transitions of valence electrons. For the greatest quantitative sensitivity (greatest absorbance change per unit of concentration), the wavelength of greatest absorption is chosen. This selection would be tempered by the consideration of potential measurement errors, which are introduced either by variations in instrument use (e.g., reproducing wavelength settings) or by the presence of interfering compounds that absorb in the same region. A broad absorption peak may be preferable to a narrow one of slightly greater height, particularly for wide–band pass instruments. Occasionally a wavelength on the shoulder of the absorption peak may be used to intentionally reduce the sensitivity of the method as a compromise to gain an increased range of linearity on the standard curve. The pitfall in this technique is the necessity for accurate wavelength settings in order to retain reproducibility in the results. In practice, the problem can be circumvented by including appropriate standards with each analysis.

■ **What is dark current?**

When two electrodes of a photodetector are maintained at different electrical potentials (i.e., have a voltage across them), they tend to "leak" electrons, producing a small flow of current even in the absence of stimulating light. Since this current does not represent the measurement of light radiation, it would introduce an error if it were added to the true photocurrent; therefore, it is neutralized by a variable resistance (the zero adjustment).

■ **What instrument component failures would produce instability at zero %T in the spectrophotometer? At 100%T?**

Instability (fluctuation) at zero suggests a weak or defective amplifier tube. Sustained drifting (in one direction) may implicate the power supply. Instability at 100%T, but not at zero, suggests an unstable light source (or power supply) or a noisy or failing photodetector.

■ **What would you conclude from the inability to set 100%T at the lower extreme of the visible region (tungsten light source)?**

The tungsten lamp emits only a small amount of radiation in the violet portion of the spectrum, its peak emission being in the infrared region. Consequently, the detector sensitivity, amplifier gain, and light source emission must all be in respectable condition for adequate operation at this end of the spectrum. This problem most likely indicates that the source lamp has deteriorated. The spectral output curve of an incandescent lamp shifts toward the infrared region, producing even less ultraviolet light as it ages. Other possible, though less likely, causes include an aging photodetector or a weak amplifier due to a component failure.

■ **How can the accuracy of the spectrophotometer's wavelength calibration be verified?**

Although the exact procedure depends on the capability of the instrument in question, the general philosophy is the same. Since the emission line spectra of some lamps (e.g., hydrogen, mercury, helium) and the absorption spectra of pure compounds (didymium and holmium oxide) are characteristic of the material, an instrument in calibration should be able to confirm these established wavelength peaks. Generally, a prism instrument should be checked at several points, since the prism dispersion is not linear, although two points may be adequate for a grating instrument. Wide–band pass instruments commonly used in routine colorimetric methods can be checked with any reproducible colored solution with a characteristic absorption peak (e.g., cobalt chloride, nickel sulfate).

■ **What is an isosbestic point?**

Since the absorption spectrum of a compound is intimately related to the structure of its molecule, it is not surprising that different forms of the same compound will have absorption peaks at different wavelengths. The isosbestic point is a wavelength where all equilibrium forms of the molecule have the same absorptivity (absorbance per unit of concentration), so quantitative measurements using this wavelength will be independent of the changes in the chemical equilibrium. This principle is used in several hemoglobinometers (using 548.5 nm) and oximeters on the market.

■ **What is the difference between a total consumption burner and a premix type?**

The total consumption burner aspirates sample directly into the base of the flame. The oxidant enters the flame at high velocity through a path concentric to that of the sample capillary. The high velocity of the oxidant produces an area of reduced pressure over the capillary. All of the sample drawn into the capillary by the partial vacuum is sheared into fine droplets and consumed in the flame. In the premix configuration, the stream of oxidant passes perpendicularly over the sample capillary and throws the resulting mist against the wall of the atomizer chamber. Most of the droplets flow down the wall and out the waste drain. The remaining finest droplets are combined with the fuel in the upper part of the chamber before the final mixture is injected into the burner. Most recent atomizer-burners are of the premix configuration.

■ **What is the internal standard technique in flame photometry and why is lithium the most common choice?**

In theory, the emission of light in the flame is directly proportional to the concentration of the element in the flame. In practice, several factors modify this ideal relationship and result in differing emission values for the same amount of sample. The internal standard technique incorporates a known constant amount of the standard element in the diluent. The diluent is used for all samples and calibrating solutions. The instrument simultaneously monitors the emission of the standard and each test element through separate photodetectors and calculates the sample concentrations on the basis of electronic comparison with the standard.

Lithium is chosen as the standard for sodium and potassium determinations for two reasons: (1) lithium emission characteristics are sufficiently similar to those of sodium and potassium so that conditions that would produce variations in emission of the test elements would produce similar changes in the lithium emission; and (2) lithium is normally a trace element in human tissues and does not present interference. Current use of lithium salts in psychiatric therapy has modified the second condition and generated a clinical demand for lithium determinations, since lithium is toxic above about 2 mEq/liter in serum. Several recent flame photometers are equipped for lithium determinations and use potassium as the internal standard.

■ **Distinguish the principles of flame emission and atomic absorption photometry.**

When a solution is evaporated in a flame, the salt crystals are vaporized and the cations reduced to their neutral electronic state. The electrons of the neutral atom can be excited to higher energy states by absorbing specific amounts of energy. In flame photometry this absorbed energy comes from the heat of the flame. When these unstable excited electrons return to their original ground state, they emit exactly the same quantity of energy that was required to reach the excited condition. In both techniques the central unifying concept is that a given electronic transition requires a very specific quanta of energy to raise the energy state, and the transition downward liberates the same quanta of energy. Light can be the form of energy involved in these transitions. The quantity of energy in a beam of light is inversely related to the wavelength. Therefore, a given electronic transition always involves the same wavelength of light. Flame emission photometry quantitates the number of atoms present in the flame as a function of the light emitted by the small percentage of atoms that become excited and return to ground state. Atomic absorption measures the much more numerous neutral atoms in the flame as a function of their ability to absorb light energy. The wavelength of light absorbed is identical to that emitted in the case of flame photometry, since the identical electronic transition is involved. In atomic absorption, whether or not the excited atom returns to ground state and emits light is unimportant.

■ **List the basic components of a simple fluorometer.**

The basic components of a simple fluorometer are (1) a source of exciting radiation—generally in the ultraviolet region; (2) a primary monochromator to isolate the exciting wavelength—an absorption filter is the simplest; (3) a cuvette to hold the sample; (4) a secondary monochromator to isolate the wavelength of fluorescence emission while blocking any stray radiation from the exciting beam; (5) a photodetector to measure the fluorescence emission—usually a photomultiplier, since the intensity of fluorescence is quite low (NOTE: The path of exciting radiation and the path from the sample to the detector are commonly placed perpendicular to avoid detecting interfering emission of the source); and (6) a readout system.

■ **What is a glass electrode and how does it measure pH?**

The glass electrode for pH measurement consists of an internal reference electrode (e.g., silver/silver chloride) submerged in a solution of known pH and enclosed in a glass bulb of special pH-sensitive glass. The sensitive glass is usually fused to a barrel of high-resistance glass that is not pH sensitive in order to avoid measurement errors from varying depths of immersion. The special glass develops a potential difference between its two surfaces that is proportional to the difference between the pH values of the test solution and the internal solution. The potential must be measured using a second reference electrode immersed in the test solution and an electronic voltmeter with very high input impedance.

■ **Describe two common types of reference electrodes for pH measurement.**

Two reference electrodes are (1) calomel (mercury chloride) electrode, which consists of an inert lead-in wire (e.g., platinum) in contact with a paste of mercury and mercury chloride and surrounded by a solution of KCl saturated with calomel; and (2) silver/silver chloride electrode, which consists of a metallic silver wire coated with a layer of silver chloride and surrounded by a solution of KCl saturated with silver chloride. In both cases, electrical contact with the test solution is accomplished by a salt bridge of KCl.

■ **How does the Severinghaus CO_2 electrode measure P_{CO_2}?**

The CO_2 electrode consists of a combination pH electrode immersed in a buffer solution of $KHCO_3$ and covered with a gas-permeable membrane (e.g., Teflon). Carbon dioxide gas diffuses across the membrane at a rate proportional to its partial pressure in the sample. The interaction of CO_2 (as carbonic acid) and $KHCO_3$ results in a change in pH, which can be measured directly with the pH electrode and electronically related to the P_{CO_2}.

■ **How does a P_{O_2} electrode work?**

The principle is based on the technique of polarography. The electrode consists of a platinum cathode and a tubular silver anode that are electrically connected by an electrolyte filling solution at their tips. The entire sensing tip is covered with a gas-permeable membrane. The electrodes are maintained at a constant potential of about 0.8 V. The oxygen diffuses across the membrane at a rate proportional to its partial pressure in the sample and is reduced at the cathode. The oxidation product, silver oxide, is subsequently formed at the silver anode. The small current produced as a result of this exchange of electrons is measured by an electrometer and can be electronically related to the P_{O_2}.

■ **What does the slope control on a pH meter actually adjust?**

The pH meter measures pH as a function of the potential difference (voltage) between the two electrodes. If the actual millivolt response of the system is plotted against the pH of known buffers, the slope of the line produced represents the millivolt change per pH unit. The slope control adjusts this response to the theoretic (Nernst) value of 59.16 mV/pH unit at 25° C. Since the response is linear, the slope can be set by calibrating the meter at any second pH value (e.g., pH 4.01) after calibration at midrange (i.e., pH 7.0).

■ **Why are both voltage and current levels of interest in electrophoresis?**

Electrophoresis separates proteins on the basis of their differences in net electrical charge. The rate of migration in an electric field is directly related to the applied voltage. Higher voltages produce faster separations and generally better resolution. The amount of current that flows in the system is a significant indication of the amount of heat that is generated and must be successfully dissipated to avoid distortions of pattern, denaturation of protein, or drying of the support medium. High current should be avoided, because the power (heat) dissipation increases as the square of the current.

■ **Describe the coulombetric method for chloride determination.**

Chloride ions are titrated ion-for-ion with Ag^+ that is generated electronically by a constant current source and a pair of silver wire electrodes. The titration product, AgCl, is essentially insoluble, and the endpoint is detected amperometrically at a second pair of electrodes by the sudden increased current due to excess Ag^+. The number of chloride ions in the sample is equal to the number of Ag^+ ions generated and is quantitatively related to the time required for the titration as follows:

$$Ag^0 \text{ (anode)} \rightarrow Ag^+ + e^-$$
$$6.24 \times 10^{18} \text{ } e^- = 1 \text{ coulomb of charge}$$
$$1 \text{ amp (constant current source)} = 1 \text{ coulomb/sec}$$

Therefore: 1 second of titration at 1 amp corresponds to
6.24×10^{18} chloride ions

■ **What is the principle of the Coulter Company's cell-counting devices?**

A suitable dilution of cells is prepared in an electrolyte solution and a known volume of the dilution is drawn through an aperture of small diameter (e.g., 100μ). A constant regulated current is maintained between two platinum electrodes placed on either side of the electrolyte-filled aperture. The cells are poor electrical conductors themselves, but they displace their volume of electrolyte as they pass through the aperture. The increased resistance (or decreased conductivity) to current flow results in a momentary pulse representing the increased voltage drop across the aperture as the cell passes through the orifice. The instrument recognizes and counts the cells as electrical pulses. The instrument can electronically discriminate cells of a selected size, since the pulse size is directly proportional to the cell size. Coincidence losses caused by simultaneous passage of more than one cell through the aperture can be predicted statistically and thus corrected according to the total number of cells counted in the aliquot.

■ **What is the function of the mercury manometer in the Coulter counter?**

The mercury column is unbalanced when vacuum is momentarily applied to one end. As it returns to its equilibrium position, it syphons the diluted cell suspension through the aperture at a uniform rate. The mercury, being electrically conductive, is also used as a switching device to control the counting section of the instrument. Three electrodes (start, stop, and common) are implanted in the wall of the mercury-filled manometer tubing in contact with the mercury. The volume displaced by the mercury between the start and stop signals is exactly 0.5 ml. The cell suspension is drawn through the aperture during the entire time the mercury column is in motion, but the instrument counts only the cells in the aliquot predetermined by the position of the start and stop electrodes.

■ **What is another principle used in automated cell-counting devices?**

Generally, it involves an optical system, although there are considerable variations. The cell suspension is passed through a flow cuvette positioned in a light beam, and the light is scattered by the cells that pass through the beam. The illumination of the cells may be direct (bright field) or indirect (dark field). The illuminated cells are viewed by a photodetector, and the number of light flashes are counted. Cell sizes are discriminated by light intensity, and the threshold settings regulate the sensitivity of the photodetector.

One company is currently marketing an optical cell counter using a "soft" laser and a unique flow-chamber design.

■ **Which values are actually measured on the Coulter model S (Sr) and which are calculated by the computer?**

RBC count, WBC count, hemoglobin, and MCV (from summated RBC volume) are actually measured. From these values the remainder are calculated: hematocrit, MCH, and MCHC.

■ **What is the purpose of air segmentation in Technicon's continuous-flow principle of automated analysis?**

In continuous-flow analysis, all samples are carried through the same analysis pathway, and the accuracy of the methodology hinges on minimizing sample interaction—in other words, the previous sample must be adequately washed out to avoid affecting the results of subsequent samples. Without air segmentation, fluid flow through the tubing is streamlined; the layers nearest the tubing wall move more slowly than the fluid in the center. The result of this outer layer hanging back is contamination of the samples that follow. Air segmentation is used to greatly reduce washing time between samples. The surface tension at the air/fluid interface holds the liquid segment together and leaves only a very thin wetting layer on the tubing wall after the segment has passed.

■ **How is protein removed from samples in the autoanalyzer system?**

The autoanalyzer uses dialysis to separate soluble chemical constituents from the proteins in a nondestructive manner. The diluted sample (usually serum) and the recipient reagent flow in parallel pathways that are separated by a semipermeable membrane. Proteins, because they are in the size range of colloidal particles, cannot diffuse through the membrane along with the truly dissolved substances, and so they are left behind. Dialysis occurs in both directions but is never carried to completion. Preheating of the dialyzing streams and constant temperature control are essential to reproducible dialysis and to the accuracy of the test result.

■ **Most automated systems other than those of the Technicon company are described as "discrete analysis" systems. What does this mean?**

In discrete systems, each sample reaction is handled in a separate compartment and does not come into contact with another sample. The exact physical arrangement of the system has several variations: individual sets of tubes that are washed before the next sample is introduced, or disposable reaction vessels, or even individual packages that contain all the required premeasured reagents. In some cases, these packages are used as the cuvette for reading colorimetric reactions.

■ **What is a potentiometric recorder and how does it work?**

A potentiometer is a device used to accurately measure voltage (electrical potential) by a null-balance technique. The unknown voltage is introduced into the potentiometer circuit so that it opposes (in polarity) a known reference voltage. The value of the unknown is measured by comparison to determine the voltage required to exactly oppose the flow of current in the test circuit. This same principle is incorporated in the potentiometric recorder to produce a continuously balancing null-point instrument with a written record. The input signal is compared with the reference signal in a differential amplifier. If the signals are not identical, the difference (error voltage) is amplified sufficiently to drive a servomotor attached to a recording pen and slidewire resistor. Any fraction of the reference voltage may be selected for comparison by moving the sliding contact to the proper point on the slidewire. The servomotor (L., slave) simply seeks out the null-balance point on the slidewire by trial and error voltage.

■ **How is the photomultiplier tube used to detect gamma radiation?**

The photomultiplier detects light flashes produced when gamma radiation is absorbed by a scintillator material and emitted as a pulse of visible or ultraviolet light. The scintillator may be a crystal attached directly to the photomultiplier envelope or a liquid in which the sample is dispersed.

■ **What is analog information?**

Information that is electronically represented as a varying voltage or current is said to be analog in nature. The signal is an electrical analogy representing the varying input parameter (e.g., light intensity, pressure, temperature). Meters and gauges are examples of analog-type readout devices that translate the signals into a physical displacement of the indicator needle.

■ **What is digital information?**

Information represented as discrete integers is referred to as digital information. A digital computer electronically represents data as individual numbers (binary) and actually solves problems by doing simple arithmetic. Digital readout devices on laboratory instruments display the result (e.g., %T or concentration units) as integers and may eliminate reading errors possible with meter scales. Analog-to-digital converters are circuits that can convert the former electrical signal into the latter for the readout device or a computer interface.

■ **What is meant by the terms "hardware" and "software"?**

Computer hardware refers to the mechanical and electrical components of a computer system. Computer software is the set of codes and instructions (i.e., programs) required to make the computer system operate.

■ **Distinguish between the terms "on-line" and "off-line."**

These terms describe the relationship between a terminal or interfaced laboratory instrument and the computer central processing unit (CPU). If the communication is direct, the relationship is said to be on-line. If the data from the terminal or instrument are collected and temporarily stored (e.g., on punched cards, magnetic tape, or punched paper tape) and must be brought to the computer by the user, the relationship is described as off-line. When an instrument is said to be interfaced with the computer, it implies that information is transmitted to the computer (on-line) or temporary data storage (off-line) without human intervention.

■ **What is a bit?**

Digital computers perform operations on information coded as discrete integers based on the binary number system. A bit is the smallest piece of information that the computer deals with—the BInary digiT (either 1 or 0).

■ **What is meant by machine language and alphanumeric language?**

Machine language is the binary-coded information that the computer actually understands and uses to perform its operations. Alphanumeric language is any language that contains both letters (alphabet) and numerals. Computer programs are more easily understood by the user when represented in the mnemonic shorthand, called assembly language, which is alphanumeric and closer to standard English.

■ **What is a CRT?**

A cathode ray tube (CRT) is a special form of vacuum tube that can visually display electrical information. It is the "picture tube" of the oscilliscope monitor and the computer terminal display. It consists of an electron gun, which projects a beam of electrons onto a phosphor-coated screen (also the tube's anode), and several electrodes to control the focus, intensity, and position of the beam. The beam can be moved across the screen to produce pictures, waveforms, and alphanumeric displays by using appropriate electrical signals on the horizontal and vertical deflection electrodes.

■ **Describe two systems for clot detection in coagulation instruments.**

In principle, any of the changes resulting from clot formation can be used to establish the time of coagulation: changes in viscosity or fluidity, optical transparency, or electrical conductivity. Two techniques commonly used at present are electrical conductivity and transparency. The latter method claims the advantage that no foreign material need be in contact with the test plasma to potentially influence coagulation.

■ **What is the principle of osmolality measurement used in most osmometers?**

Any of the four interrelated colligative properties resulting when any substance is dissolved in a solvent could in theory be used to determine the number of particles in solution and thus the molality: (1)

depression of the freezing point, (2) elevation of the boiling point, (3) decrease in the vapor pressure, or (4) increase in the osmotic pressure.

Most instruments measure the depression of the freezing point (compared with that of the pure solvent). The instrument consists of a refrigeration unit, a stirring probe, a thermistor to measure the temperature, a constant current source, and a wheatstone-bridge balancing circuit. In operation, the sample is rapidly cooled below its freezing point without ice formation (supercooling), and freezing of the unstable liquid is initiated by mechanical shock from the stirring probe. As the supercooled liquid freezes, the formation of crystals liberates heat and the temperature of the sample rises to its true freezing point. The freezing point is measured by the thermistor and the wheatstone-bridge circuit during the equilibrium period, which lasts until freezing is complete. A thermistor is a temperature-sensitive resistor made of transition metal oxides.

■ **What two methods can be used to verify the accuracy of an autodilutor?**

The accuracy of both sample aspiration and diluent delivery can be determined gravimetrically using water in preweighed vials. Generally, an average value of several aspirations or deliveries is determined. If the dilution ratio is the major concern, the results of macrodilutions with volumetric glassware can be compared with those of the dilutor using spectrophotometry. A dye such as ferroin (phenanthroline ferrous sulfate complex), which absorbs at 508 nm and follows Beer's law over a wide range of concentration, is used as the sample to be diluted.

■ **List the basic components of a gas-liquid chromatograph.**

The basic components of a gas-liquid chromatograph are: (1) injection port, (2) column, (3) column oven, including temperature controls, (4) detector, including temperature controls, (5) electrometer or power supply (depending on detector type), and (6) recorder.

■ **List three types of detectors for gas chromatography.**

Three types of detectors for gas chromatography are: (1) thermal conductivity detector, (2) flame ionization detector, and (3) electron capture detector.

■ **What is the basic principle of separations by gas-liquid chromatography (GLC)?**

Any material that is volatile or can be converted into a volatile derivative can be analyzed by GLC. The separation is based on the difference in solubility of the material between the carrier gas phase and the inert liquid phase coated on the column walls or packing. The sample is vaporized at the injection port and swept into the column by the carrier gas. The sample components partition themselves between the two phases on the basis of their individual diffusion rates and their relative solubilities in the liquid phase. The result is that components move through the column at different rates and appear at different times at the detector. The time of retention in the column is characteristic of the sample component and the analysis conditions and is rarely identical for two compounds. Passage through the detector generates an analog signal that is recorded on a moving chart. The component can be identified by its retention time in comparison with that of an internal standard and can be quantitated by integration of the peak area. The gas chromatograph can be interfaced with a mass spectrometer to provide the ultimate in sample separation and identification.

■ **Distinguish between the terms "accuracy" and "precision."**

Accuracy describes how closely an experimental result approaches the true value of the quantity being measured. Precision describes the reproducibility of repeated measurements on the same sample and is an indication of the cumulative effect of all random experimental errors inherent in the procedure. It is easily possible for a method to yield precise results and to be entirely inaccurate.

■ **What is the purpose of quality control in the clinical laboratory?**

Quality control programs are designed to assure that laboratory results are reliable, that is, both accurate and precise, on a day-to-day basis.

■ **What is the place of statistical evaluation in the quality control program?**

Since repeated analysis on the same sample (e.g., a control sample) will generally not give identical results, the significance of the cumulative contributions to random error in the method can be adequately evaluated only by statistical methods. A graphic plotting of a series of replicate results versus the frequency of occurrence of each value would produce a normal, bell-shaped (gaussian) curve with the average value (arithmetic mean) in the center and with approximately half of the values lower and the other half higher than the mean. With a sufficiently large number of aliquots, the mean value will closely approach the true value of the constituent being measured—i.e., averaging the results reduces the chance of any one result being erroneous. The precision of the method is indicated by the standard deviation, which is a measure of the scatter of values around the mean. The smaller the standard deviation, the greater the precision. Laboratory results are said to be in statistical control when the significant sources of error are known and kept under control as indicated by the results of routine quality control samples, which fall within the prescribed acceptable limits established by statistical evaluation.

■ **Why should a quality control specimen closely resemble the patient samples both chemically and physically?**

The underlying premise is that any patient sample is subject to a series of random experimental errors throughout the course of an analysis. The highest degree of quality control is obtained when control samples are subject to all the same possible errors. Steps in the analysis that may be taken for granted, such as aspiration of the sample in an automated system or protein removal (which an aqueous control would bypass), may remain undisclosed sources of erratic results. The levels and varieties of chemical constituents should be comparable to the expected patient values. This will reproduce constant sources of chemical interference as they would be found in an actual patient sample. Note that more complete quality control is obtained by using two different controls representing both normal and pathologic levels.

■ **What is the significance of a single control value that falls outside the established limits of acceptability?**

Any control sample outside acceptable limits should be evaluated carefully before test results can be reported. Inherent in the statistical design of the quality control limits, which are defined in terms of standard deviation (SD) from the mean, is the fact that a known percentage of individual values will fall outside. For example, if the acceptable limits of a procedure are set as the mean ±2 SD, we can be statistically confident that this interval encloses 95% of the values that would be obtained by repeated analysis of the control sample. The 95% confidence level also assures us that 5%, or 1 out of 20 results, will be outside these limits and do not indicate any problem in the analysis conditions. The crux of the matter in evaluating an individual result that falls outside the limits is to determine whether this represents a true problem or is simply the 1 in 20 we should expect. If no analysis problem is obvious, we would approach the dilemma by selecting a new control sample and repeating the analysis on it as well as on several patient samples chosen at random from those that have already been run. If the new control value is now within limits and the patient values are confirmed, we can assume that the procedure is still in control. Even though the control value has been explained, both values should be recorded on the quality control chart. If the new control is still outside the limits, it may indicate a serious problem, and the analysis must be scrutinized step by step.

■ **What is the significance of a trend or shift in a quality control chart?**

From the normal frequency distribution curve (bell-shaped curve) of statistics, we should expect daily values to vary from the mean so that, on the average, half the values are above and half the values are below the mean.

Control values that show a sustained increase or decrease over several days exhibit a trend away from the mean. The trend may indicate deterioration in reagents, instrumentation, or even the control sample pool, and it must be investigated.

Control values that appear to be distributed on one side of the mean over several days may have taken a shift and should also arouse suspicion and be investigated.

■ **Is quality control necessary with automated instrument systems?**

Absolutely! Not only should controls be run daily on such systems, they should be interspersed through each batch of samples. One of the desirable qualities of automation may be the increased speed and precision with which the system can repeat manipulations, but the increased complexity of operations provides more sources of error from miscalibration. An inadequately supervised instrument will continue to produce results as long as you let it, but accuracy to accompany the precision may be entirely accidental.

CHAPTER 8

Chemistry

This chapter is both review and overview. You are reminded to return to your (perhaps dusty) biochemistry textbook and to clinical texts containing specific methodologies for details that you may have forgotten or have not as yet fully appreciated. We hope that this overview will refresh your memory, tie together loose ends, and perhaps provide a perspective to the applications of undergraduate chemistry.

Lipids, proteins, and carbohydrates
JOAN SHROUT

■ **What are the plasma lipids?**

Plasma lipids include phospholipids; sterols such as cholesterol and cholesterol esters; mono-, di-, and triglycerides; and nonesterified fatty acids. Total lipid analysis also includes fat-soluble vitamins.

■ **Give the general functions of plasma lipids in the body.**

In general, lipids are required as components of cellular and subcellular membranes (phospholipid, cholesterol), as a source of energy to tissue, as components for other substances (cholesterol for steroid hormones and vitamins, phospholipid for thromboplastin), as insulation and padding for organs, and as components for neural myelin sheaths.

■ **Where and how does lipid synthesis occur?**

Most of the endogenous plasma lipids are synthesized by the liver, the overall metabolic pathway having many steps.

The exogenous lipid molecules are ingested and broken down to varying degrees in the intestine by the bile acids and pancreatic secretions (e.g., lipase). Chylomicrons are formed in the intestinal cells and, via the lymphatics and systemic circulation, go to adipose tissue, where they are either hydrolyzed or resynthesized, or to the liver.

In the liver the exogenous molecules are disassembled and then rebuilt (as demonstrated by radioactive tagging). Synthesis of protein also occurs in the liver, and normally the "rebuilt" lipids are conjugated with a specific protein forming the lipoprotein.

Lipids can be acquired exogenously from the diet or can be derived endogenously. The latter is especially true of cholesterol, which can be synthesized from acetate groups in most organ tissues.

■ **What are lipoproteins and how are they classified?**

Lipoproteins are lipid-protein complexes (about 30% protein) that function in the transport of lipids.

Electrophoretically, the lipoprotein mobilities match those of the globulins, leading to classification as alpha-, prebeta-, and beta-lipoproteins. Chylomicrons are detected by electrophoresis as a nonmigrating band at the point of origin, although serum from a fasting patient should normally reveal no chylomicron band. Normally, the alpha complex is the principal carrier of phospholipid (30%); the prebeta complex carries mainly triglyceride (44%) and some cholesterol (18%); the beta complex is the chief carrier of cholesterol (43%) as well as albumin, which transports the fatty acids.

By ultracentrifugation, the lipoproteins are separated into very low-density lipoprotein (VLDL, prebeta), low-density lipoprotein (LDL, beta), and high-density lipoprotein (HDL, alpha).

■ **What are sources of error encountered in lipid-profile testing?**

Lipid testing must be performed after the patient has fasted for 12 to 14 hours. The patient should be on a normal diet 7 days before testing. Lipoprotein studies should not be performed for 6 weeks after myocardial infarct. Care should be taken to prevent bacterial contamination of the blood specimen, because this may lead to unclear electrophoretic pattern as well as to possible increase in triglycerides and increased anodic migration of beta and prebeta bands. (Add 1.5% thimerosal to serum to prevent bacterial growth.) Specimens should not be frozen, because this may also lead to loss of clear bands. Lipid abnormalities can be of two classes: hypolipidemia, a decrease in one or more lipoproteins or lipids (e.g., abetalipoproteinemia, Tangier disease), or hyperlipidemia, an increase in one or more lipoproteins or lipids.

■ **What is lipid phenotyping?**

Phenotyping is the classification of hyperlipidemias into five main types. The classification is based on ultracentrifugation results, or the electrophoretic pattern of serum, in agreement with specific lipid fraction tests, especially of cholesterol and triglyceride. Each of the five types has a characteristic pattern of increases in specific lipids and lipoproteins (Table 9).

Table 9. Predominant characteristics found in each of the five types of hyperlipidemia (classification of Fredrickson, Levy, and Lees)

	Description	Lipid pattern	Serum	Other
Type I	Familial fat-induced hyperlipidemia Rare	Chylomicrons present Triglycerides increased Cholesterol increased (usually)	Turbid; creamy supernatant with clear infranate	Deficiency of lipoprotein lipase Alpha and beta fractions reduced, no prebeta
Type IIA	Familial hyperbetalipoproteinemia Common	Increased beta band; cholesterol markedly increased Normal prebeta	Clear	
Type IIB	Familial hyperbetalipoproteinemia Common	Increased beta band; cholesterol markedly increased Increased prebeta band; slight moderate increase in triglyceride; LDL ratio >190 mg/dl	Slightly turbid without chylomicron layer	
Type III	Familial hyperbeta- and prebetalipoproteinemia Uncommon, but not rare	Abnormal beta (low density, <1.006 gm/ml) with high amount of cholesterol Increase in S_f 12-20 and S_f 20-100 Cholesterol and triglyceride increased, cholesterol > triglyceride	Turbid	Abnormal glucose tolerance Only genetic causes°
Type IV	Carbohydrate-induced hyperlipemia Common	Distinct prebeta band; increased triglyceride Normal or slightly increased cholesterol; LDL ratio <190 mg/dl	Turbid or clear	Abnormal glucose tolerance Obesity
Type V	Familial hyperchylomicronemia Rare	High levels of chylomicrons and prebeta Cholesterol increased Triglycerides increased	Turbid; creamy supernatant with lipemic infranate	Abnormal glucose tolerance

°The other types listed can occur secondary to other disorders (e.g., liver disease, pancreatitis), which must be carefully considered in regard to treatment of the lipidemia.

■ **What are the major plasma proteins?**

Identified by electrophoretic separation on cellulose acetate, the plasma proteins are albumin, alpha-1-globulins, alpha-2-globulins, beta globulins, and gamma globulins.

■ **What are the general functions of plasma proteins in the body?**

Ingested proteins can be broken down into amino acids and subsequently resynthesized into required body proteins. Amino acids are utilized to build muscle tissue and to synthesize enzymes and hormones. Proteins are the principal transport system in the body. Water-insoluble lipids, drugs, hormones, and many cations are carried by specific proteins. Proteins, especially albumin, contribute to maintenance of normal osmotic pressure and water distribution.

■ **Where is the site of protein synthesis?**

The plasma proteins are synthesized in the liver, with the exception of the gamma globulins and some beta globulins. Because of this, the albumin/globulin (A/G) ratio and tests based on it—cephalin flocculation, thymol turbidity—were developed to detect liver damage. The gamma globulins are synthesized and transported by lymphocytes (B-cells) and plasma cells. Some beta globulins are made elsewhere in the reticuloendothelial system.

The liver is also the major site for breakdown of protein. Some amino acids return to the "amino acid pool." Others undergo breakdown: through a series of reactions, ammonia is formed and then converted to urea nitrogen (in the liver). The blood urea nitrogen (BUN) is normally cleared by the kidney.

■ **Discuss the purpose of the oral glucose tolerance test and the characteristic insulin response patterns in diabetic, hypoglycemic, and "normal" individuals.**

The glucose tolerance test measures the rate of removal of a specific carbohydrate—glucose—from the bloodstream. The rate at which glucose is absorbed in the gastrointestinal tract and the rate and degree of filtration and reabsorption by the kidney are factors that may influence the tolerance curve. Malabsorption syndrome (in the intestine) or hypothyroidism can occur, resulting in a "flat" curve. Low or normal plasma glucose levels with glucose in the urine may indicate a condition called renal glycosuria.

In the normal individual the insulin response to an oral glucose load is almost immediate, with the insulin level peaking between 30 and 60 minutes. This results in the plasma glucose level peaking between 30 and 60 minutes and returning to normal limits within 3 hours.

In "maturity onset" diabetes the secretion of insulin is delayed, followed by a slightly higher than normal level at 2 hours. The blood glucose level is therefore usually elevated until around the 2-hour point. In overt diabetes there is little or no secretion of insulin, resulting in abnormally elevated glucose levels throughout the testing.

Hypoglycemia is characterized by delayed secretion of insulin followed by hypersecretion, which is believed to be the effect of prolonged stimulation of the pancreas by the increased glucose. The blood glucose level is usually below normal after the 2-hour point, through 4 and 5 hours, because of the high insulin levels.

There are various criteria to evaluate tolerance results. One commonly used is a point system (Wilkerson), with the fasting and 3-hour specimen results worth 1 point each if the result (glucose in mg/dl) is above normal limits, and the 1-hour and 2-hour results each worth ½ point if abnormally high. A score of 2 or greater indicates diabetes mellitus.

■ **What are sources of error in glucose tolerance testing?**

Incorrect preparation of the patient can lead to erroneous results. The patient must be fasting and must be given a glucose load calculated for his body mass. Also, the patient must have eaten adequate carbohydrates (150 gm/day) for 72 hours before testing. The patient should not have been subjected to recent trauma (surgery, myocardial infarct, labor and delivery, and so on).

■ **Which hormones contribute to the regulation of the blood glucose level?**

Two hormones directly regulate the blood glucose. Glucagon and insulin are both produced in the pancreas, in the alpha and beta cells of the islet of Langerhans, respectively. The secretion of glucagon accelerates the breakdown of glycogen (glycogenolysis) in the liver, causing an increase in blood glucose. Secretion of insulin results in an increased permeability of certain cellular membranes to glucose. It further stimulates formation of glycogen from glucose in the liver, thereby reducing blood glucose levels.

Other hormones also contribute to glucose metabolism. ACTH and growth hormone from the pituitary, 11-oxy-21 steroids from the adrenal cortex, epinephrine from the adrenal medulla, and thyroxine from the thyroid exert effects on the metabolic pathways of glucose.

■ **List other carbohydrate tolerance tests.**

Tolerance tests can also be performed for pentoses, lactose, galactose and D-xylose.

■ **What is the purpose of a tolbutamide tolerance test?**

Tolbutamide (Orinase) is a hypoglycemic agent that acts by stimulating the pancreatic beta cells to produce insulin. Delayed or low production of insulin occurs in some adult individuals and is termed "maturity onset" diabetes. The glucose levels after tolbutamide stimulation have distinctive patterns as compared with nondiabetic response to tolbutamide. Abnormal response to this tolerance test can also indicate adenoma of the pancreas.

■ **What is the significance of lactic acid?**

Lactic acid is a metabolite of anaerobic glucose metabolism within the muscle tissue (tricarboxylic acid cycle). Strenuous exercise or muscle trauma will result in elevated lactate levels. Normally, this is removed (detoxified) by the liver. In liver dysfunction, however, the blood lactate level rises. Decreased cardiac output (e.g., congestive heart failure) may also contribute to rising lactate levels because of decreased oxygen delivery to the tissues.

•　•　•

Table 10 lists the reference methods for some test analyses commonly performed in clinical chemistry. The exact methods and procedures can be found in textbooks. It is of some importance to be acquainted with the reference method in terms of understanding inherent error, e.g., measurement of glucose on the autoanalyzer versus

Table 10. Reference methods as well as one or two of the commonly performed procedures for tests discussed in this chapter

Test	Reference method	Routine clinical method
Total lipid	Sperry and Brand; gravimetric	Phosphovanillin
Cholesterol	Abell; gravimetric	Lieberman-Burchard
Triglyceride	Van Handel; gravimetric; glycerol determination with phospholipid removed by zeolite	Glycerol determination with Hantzsche (acetylacetone) color reaction
		Enzymatic
Total protein	Kjeldahl; gravimetric; determination of protein nitrogen	Biuret
Glucose	Hexokinase, enzymatic; glucose oxidase, enzymatic (although inhibitors may be present)	Alkaline ferricyanide; cupric neocuprine
Calcium	Atomic absorption	8-OH-quinoline
		Atomic absorption
Chloride	Schales and Schales; titration with mercuric nitrate	Cotlove chloridometers

"true glucose" values. Although this discrepancy does not routinely produce problems in the clinical laboratory, the technologist should be aware of the existence of such discrepancy or variance among methods and should have some concept of the underlying reasons for the variance.

Hormones and enzymes

ANTHONY CAFARO

In the following discussion, enzymes will be named and abbreviated in accordance with the recommendations of the Commission on Enzymes of the International Unit on Biochemistry. Most notable are the following.

Recommended name and abbreviation	*Common name and abbreviation*
Alkaline phosphatase (ALP)	Alkaline phosphatase (ALP)
Alanine transaminase (ALT)	Glutamic pyruvic transaminase (GPT)
Aspartate transaminase (AST)	Glutamic oxaloacetic transaminase (GOT)
Creatine kinase (CK)	Creatine phosphokinase (CPK)
Lactate dehydrogenase (LD)	Lactic acid dehydrogenase (LDH)

■ **What is an enzyme?**

An enzyme is a protein product of living cells that catalyzes chemical reactions independent of the cell.

■ **How is the synthesis of enzymes controlled?**

Enzymes are under genetic control—one gene, one polypeptide.

■ **What is their composition?**

Enzymes have two principal components. The apoenzyme portion is protein, thermolabile, and nondialyzable; the coenzyme portion is organic, thermostable, and dialyzable.

■ **Are enzymes always immediately active after their formation?**

No. Many enzymes exist in an inactive form, referred to as a preenzyme or a proenzyme. These substances sometimes require the presence of activators, which may be ionic or nonionic. Such substances include magnesium, cobalt, manganese, hormones, catecholamines, and other enzymes.

■ **Can enzymatic action be inactivated?**

Yes. Enzymes may be inactivated both in vivo and in vitro. Substances such as cyanide, mercury, arsenicals, carbon monoxide, and certain narcotics are sulfhydryl inhibitors. In vitro inactivation is related to the protein nature of the enzyme and is principally concerned with changes in temperature and pH.

■ **Where are enzymes located within the cell?**

Enzymes may be located within the cytoplasm of the cell, within the subcellular organelles, or within the nucleus. The cytoplasmic enzymes are the most primitive and principally carry on anaerobic metabolism. This includes some of the transaminases, peptidases, and phosphorylases, as well as enzymes required for fatty acid synthesis and glycolysis. When cellular damage occurs, these enzymes are the first to appear in the serum. Lysosomes contain acid phosphatase, ribonuclease, and cathepsin. Incomplete phagocytosis occurs when these enzymes are deficient. Within the mitochondria are enzymes that are principally concerned with aerobic metabolism and are most affected by poison such as cyanide, which destroys the oxidative capacity of the cell. When these enzymes appear in increased levels in the serum, they are indicative of a more advanced degree of cellular destruction. Microsomes contain alkaline phosphatase (ALP), esterases, and enzymes for both lipid and protein synthesis. The nucleus contains enzymes for glycolysis and nucleic acid synthesis.

■ **What is the clinical significance of enzymatic localization?**

Inasmuch as similar enzymes are located in different portions of the cell, the appearance of the specific isoenzymes within the serum may denote the degree of cellular damage. For example, the aspartate transaminase (AST) is located both in the cytoplasm and within the mitochondria of the cell. The appearance of the mitochondrial fraction denotes more extensive cellular damage.

■ **How are enzymes cleared from the body?**

Different routes are used for various enzymes. Few exit via the kidney because of their relatively large molecular weight. Some are excreted via the bile, i.e., ALP and leucine aminopeptidase. Others may be destroyed intravascularly or eliminated via the gastrointestinal tract. [1,2]

■ **Can enzyme activity increase during storage?**

Yes. At refrigerator temperatures, ALP activity may increase from 10% to 30%. The enzyme, however, is stable when the sample is frozen. In contrast, acid phosphatase is very unstable; the sample should be fresh when determinations are done, or it should be separated quickly and frozen.

■ **Can hemolysis interfere with enzyme determinations?**

Yes. When hemolysis is present, lactate dehydrogenase (LD) and aldolase levels may be significantly elevated. Lesser increases are seen in the determinations of glutamyltransferase, AST, isocitrate dehydrogenase, acid phosphatase, creatine kinase (CK), leucine aminopeptidase, and alanine transaminase (ALT).

■ **Are all enzymes stable at refrigerator temperatures?**

No. Acid phosphatase is very unstable. CK activity will decrease up to 50% per day at refrigerator temperatures. Other enzymes having a half-life between 2 and 3 days are AST, ALT, LD, and glutamate dehydrogenase.

■ **How are enzymes named?**

Enzymes are named on the basis of the substrate on which they react, followed by a suffix that denotes the type of action the enzyme exerts on the substrate; for example, lactate dehydrogenase—the substrate is lactate, the function is to remove hydrogen.

■ **What is the definition of a standard unit?**

One standard unit is the amount of enzyme that catalyzes the conversion of one micromole (microequivalent) of substrate or coenzyme per minute under defined test conditions (the usual recommended temperature is 25° C). The pH is variable and must be adjusted for the optimum reactivity of the particular enzyme.

■ **What are the factors that affect enzyme activity?**

Temperature, pH, substrate concentration, and enzyme concentration all affect enzyme activity.

■ **What is the effect of temperature on an enzymatic reaction?**

The activity of most enzymes increases by a factor of 1.4 to 2 for each 10° C increment between 10° and 30° C. A temperature difference of 1° C may affect the activity by 4 % to 10%.

■ **What is the relationship between reaction rate and substrate concentration in enzyme determinations?**

In enzyme testing, the rate of the reaction should not be affected by substrate concentration; that is, the addition of more substrate will not alter the rate of enzymatic activity. This is referred to as zero order kinetics.

■ **What is meant by "first order kinetics" in enzyme determinations?**

In enzyme determinations, the term first order kinetics refers to the activity of the enzyme being proportional to its concentration; that is, the more enzyme present, the faster the reactions. All enzyme reactions should be first order kinetic with respect to enzyme concentration and zero order kinetic with respect to substrate concentration.

■ **What is the general classification of enzymes?**

A general classification of clinical enzymes includes oxidases, dehydrogenases, transferases, hydrolases, lyases, and isomerases.

■ **What is an isoenzyme?**

Isoenzymes are enzymes that react on a similar substrate but may differ in their chemical properties, i.e., pH optima and relative charge.

■ **What is the character of the LD isoenzymes and how are they designated?**

By electrophoresis, five distinct bands are identified. The most cathodic, LD fraction 5, migrates with the gamma globulins. All the other fractions migrate toward the anode. Some confusion exists regarding the nomenclature, because some people have reversed the order. In most of the literature, however, the most anodic fraction is fraction 1, which is the heart fraction; fraction 5, the liver fraction, is the slowest. In this discussion, this is the format that will be followed.

■ **How may one make an assessment of these enzymes without electrophoresis?**

This may be accomplished by measuring the total LD activity and then determining the heat-resistant fraction of LD; fraction 1 resists denaturation at 58° C for 30 minutes, whereas the activity of the other four isoenzymes is destroyed under these conditions. This may also be confirmed by an alpha-hydroxybutyrate dehydrogenase determination. The activity of this enzyme parallels that of the LD fraction 1.

■ **Are the LD and isoenzyme determinations valid after the serum has been frozen?**

No. Fractions 4 and 5 are rapidly destroyed by freezing and are diminished after storage at 4° C. Some investigators have noted that no significant alteration occurs in the activity of the isoenzymes for up to 10 days if sera are stored at room temperature.

■ **Can isoenzyme determinations of LD be performed by alternate methods?**

Yes. Biochemical-inhibition methods utilizing oxalate are used to inhibit the fast isoenzymes and methods utilizing urea to inhibit the isoenzymes of low electrophoretic mobility. Others have noted that pyruvate enhances the activity of the LD fraction 1 in the presence of urea and thus have used the LD isoenzyme index with 2 M lactate and .02 M lactate plus 2 M urea as substrate.

■ **Is there ever a clinical situation in which more than 5 LD isoenzyme bands may be seen?**

Yes. If an isoenzyme determination is performed on seminal fluid, an X band will appear having a mobility between LD fractions 3 and 4. This band is characteristic of the mature testes and is observed in seminal plasma in relation to the number of spermatozoa present; that is, if the patient is aspermic, the LD fraction X will not be present.

■ **What enzymes are clinically useful in the evaluation of myocardial disease, principally infarction?**

The enzymes that are principally concerned with evaluation of myocardial damage are LD, AST, CK, and alpha-hydroxybutyrate dehydrogenase.

■ **Is any one of the above tests totally specific for myocardial damage?**

No. All of the enzymes mentioned above may be increased in both striated muscle disease and some liver diseases.

■ **How then can one make a more useful evaluation of myocardial damage using the same enzymes?**

A more useful evaluation can be made based on isoenzyme determinations of both LD and CK. This separation of enzymes may be accomplished by electrophoresis, wherein the most anodic fractions of LD, fractions 1 and 2, are associated with myocardial damage. Both the intermediate and third fractions of CK are associated with myocardial damage.

■ **Are isoenzyme determinations helpful if the clinical history is compatible with myocardial infarction but the LD and CK determinations are normal?**

Yes. Diagnostic shifts in the isoenzyme fractionation have been noted before the clinical manifestation of abnormal increases in either of the above-mentioned enzymes is present. Therefore, when the clinical situation dictates, isoenzyme determinations may be helpful.

■ **Can one expect any single "cardiac enzyme" to be increased earlier than the others when myocardial damage is present?**

Although at various times authors have reported that CK activity is the earliest to increase, there is no hard and fast rule. Generally, in decreasing order of clinical specificity, the cardiac enzymes are related to each other as follows: LD with isoenzyme determination and CK with isoenzyme determination and hydroxybutyrate dehydrogenase. It must be remembered that LD isoenzymes and CK isoenzymes may be altered before the appearance of increased total activity.

■ **What is the specific CK isoenzyme fraction that is increased in myocardial infarction?**

CK MB. Three CK isoenzymes are recognized: BB is predominantly associated with brain tissue, MB is predominantly associated with heart tissue, and MM is present in all tissue, especially skeletal muscle. The isoenzymes may be separated by electrophoresis; however, a specific antibody to the B subunit has been developed that allows for detection of the B portion of MB. A currently reported method detects levels of B subunit in the range of 0.0001 IU/ml.[3]

■ **Can spurious increases in CK_1 (BB) be noted clinically in serum?**

Yes. Normally, only CK_3 (MM) fraction is noted in serum. However, occasionally the transient appearance of CK_1 (BB) is seen in the serum of patients who have had cardiopulmonary resuscitation following cardiac arrest, massive cerebral hemorrhage, membranous colitis, or malignancy (carcinoma of prostate).[4]

■ **Which enzymes are clinically useful in evaluating hepatic disease?**

AST, ALT, LD with isoenzyme determination, and isocitrate dehydrogenase aid in evaluating hepatic disease. When jaundice is present and the differential diagnosis of intrahepatic and extrahepatic jaundice is at issue, γ-glutamyltransferase and adenosine deaminase are of increased importance.

■ **Which enzymes are the most widely used in the clinical laboratory for the diagnosis of hepatic disease?**

The two transaminases, AST and ALT, are the most widely used.

■ **In what situations may the greatest magnitude of rise be demonstrated in the levels of these enzymes?**

In acute hepatitis and acute toxic injury to the liver, serum activity may be elevated 20 to 30 times normal.

■ **Of what use is the AST/ALT radio?**

The normal ratio is 1:1. A reversed ratio is almost always seen in acute hepatitis. In chronic hepatitis and cirrhosis, a ratio greater than 1:1 is usually noted.

■ **How many isoenzyme bands are produced on electrophoresis of AST?**

Two bands are demonstrated: a fast band, which is distributed in the cytoplasm located principally in heart and liver tissue, and a slow band, which is located in the mitochondria and seen in massive liver necrosis.

■ **What enzyme determinations are specific for liver cell necrosis?**

L-Iditol dehydrogenase (sorbitol dehydrogenase) and glutamate dehydrogenase.[5]

■ **Of what value is LD determination in liver disease?**

Total activity in the serum is nonspecific; however, fractionation of LD into isoenzymes is valuable in that an increase in the fraction 5 band is a sensitive indicator for parenchymal damage. Increases may be seen with acute parenchymal necrosis, space-occupying lesions, and congestive failure. It must be remembered that fraction 5 increases may also be seen with striated muscle injury. However, history and ALT determination are helpful in making the differential diagnosis.

■ **Can drugs have an effect on the activity of AST and LD?**

Yes. Opiates may cause a secondary increase in AST and LD by their effect on the hepatic cell. LD isoenzyme determinations will demonstrate this effect by an elevation of the level of LD fraction 5 (cathodic fraction). Also, pregnancy and oral contraceptives may cause an increase in both AST and LD.

■ **What drugs may induce liver disease?**

Two categories of drugs injurious to the liver are recognized: (1) predictable dose-related drugs such as the protoplasmic poisons (e.g., carbon tetrachloride and inorganic phosphorus), and (2) drugs that act in a somewhat more unpredictable manner, having an effect either on cell metabolism or via an idiosyncrasy of the host. Antibiotics (such as tetracycline) and antimetabolites (such as mercaptopurine) are examples of the former. Chlorpromazine is an example of the latter. Intermediate is methyl testosterone, which is toxic and also causes jaundice (cholestatic). Certain of the oral contraceptives containing testosterone derivatives can have a similar effect.

■ **Can enzymes be used to detect hepatitis when jaundice does not exist?**

Yes. Transaminases may be increased as early as 1 to 4 weeks before the clinical onset of jaundice in a patient with hepatitis. Additionally, LD isoenzyme determinations may demonstrate a prominent fraction 5 before the appearance of clinical disease.

■ **Can drugs be a cause of spurious increases in AST?**

Yes. It has been shown that PAS (para-aminosalicylic acid), a drug commonly used in the treatment of tuberculosis, can interfere with the colorimetric reaction that is sometimes used to determine AST activity. Most of these problems can be circumvented by using a reaction that requires a coenzyme such as nicotinamide adenine dinucleotide (NAD) as an intermediary reaction. The absorbance of NAD occurs in the ultraviolet range and thereby will circumvent any interfering color-producing reactions.

■ **Which enzymes are most often increased in biliary tract disease associated with cholestasis?**

The three enzymes most often associated with clinical biliary tract disease are nonspecific ALP, leucine aminopeptidase, and 5' nucleotidase.

■ **What additional information may be obtained from the determination of ALP isoenzyme?**

A significant liver band is noted on an ALP isoenzyme determination. This usually migrates in polyacrylamide gel in the area of the alpha-2 globulin. The beta-1 position is occupied by ALP of bone or placental origin, and the fraction that migrates in the beta-2 area is associated with intestinal ALP.

■ **What other enzymes are clinically useful in biliary tract disease?**

γ-Glutamyltransferase may be significantly altered in cases of obstructive jaundice.

■ **Where is γ-glutamyltransferase located and what is its clinical significance?**

γ-Glutamyltransferase is located in liver, pancreas, and kidney tissue. Its principal value is in determining the cause of jaundice. In cases of hepatocellular and obstructive jaundice, the γ-glutamyltransferase level tends to be disproportionately higher than the transaminase level. The reverse is true in viral hepatitis.

■ **Why do biliary tract enzymes increase in cases of infectious or toxic hepatitis?**

In clinical cases of hepatitis, increase in the biliary enzymes is a result of the cholestatic phase of the illness, which may be seen in both acute and chronic situations.

■ **What are some other causes for increases in the biliary tract enzymes?**

All three enzymes, ie., nonspecific ALP, 5' nucleotidase, and leucine aminopeptidase, may be increased in association with drug therapy.

■ **Which drugs are most commonly associated with cholestatic jaundice?**

Sulfonylurea derivatives are associated with cholestatic jaundice, namely, phenothiazine tranquilizers such as chlorpromazine, sulfonamides, antidiabetic drugs, and oral diuretics; anabolic steroids such as androgens; and certain of the antibiotics, principally erythromycin estolate.

■ **Can oral contraceptives (the pill) be associated with jaundice?**

Yes. Most instances of jaundice associated with the pill are seen during the first three cycles of its administration. If jaundice occurs after this time, it is believed that it most likely is not related to the pill. For this reason, it is believed that prescreening for hepatic disease should be performed before a patient is given the pill. Other interferences caused by the drug include alteration in glucose metabolism and alterations in T4 and T3 results.

■ **What enzymes are useful in the determination of muscle disease not of cardiac origin?**

CK, aldolase, and LD, particularly with isoenzyme determination, are useful determinants.

■ **Can spurious increases in these enzymes be seen?**

Yes. Increases in these enzymes may be noted following strenuous exercise. Sometimes the peak is observed between 16 and 24 hours, and the level may remain elevated for as long as 48 hours. Physical conditioning of the subject may alter the response of these enzymes.

■ **In what clinical situations may these muscle enzymes be altered?**

The most striking increases in the muscle enzymes occur in progressive Duchenne-type muscular dystrophy. It has also been noted that increases may be seen in siblings of affected children. Muscular dystrophy usually affects males, and children at age 6 months have been shown to have elevated values of these enzymes followed by the appearance of clinical signs and symptoms sometime later. Other types of dystrophies usually are associated with elevated values, but the levels are not as high as those observed in the Duchenne type.

■ **Does inflammation of the muscle cause an alteration of the muscle enzymes?**

Serum enzyme activity is associated with polymyositis syndrome; these elevations tend to parallel the severity of the disease process.

■ **Do the isoenzymes of LD in any way reflect the type of metabolism carried on in the tissue?**

Yes. Fraction 1 is generally associated with aerobic metabolism and is the type observed in cardiac muscle, whereas fraction 5 is associated with anaerobic metabolism and is observed in liver and muscle tissue.

■ **Under what clinical situations may a very high CK level not be associated with significant increases in aldolase or LD?**

When a cerebral vascular accident (stroke) or malignant hyperthermia is present, very high CK values may be noted.

■ **In what situation may a very high LD level be observed without significant increases in either aldolase or CK?**

This situation is usually seen in cases of hemolytic disease, particularly vitamin B_{12} deficiency (pernicious anemia). In this situation, the AST levels are also normal, and on isoenzyme determination of LD a very prominent fraction 1 is present.

■ **Can malignancy affect enzymes?**

Yes. Malignancies, because of multiple system involvement, may cause irregular increases in all enzymes. In these situations, there may be no characteristic pattern present unless one system is more severely affected than the others.

■ **Is there a clinical value in performing enzyme determinations on body fluids other than plasma?**

In cases of malignancy, it is advisable to perform enzyme determinations on the body fluid in question, particularly LD with isoenzyme determination. However, in these situations a concurrent serum determination should be performed, although these determinations in and of themselves are significant only if there is a notable difference between the body fluid and the serum levels, i.e., body fluid value is higher than serum value. Although no direct cause can be determined in such a situation, it does tend to support the theory that active tissue damage is occurring in the area and producing a change in the body fluid. (Body fluids refer to cerebrospinal fluid, pleural and abdominal effusions, urine, and articular fluid.)

■ **Where is ALP located?**

The ALP enzymes are ubiquitous in distribution. The primary tissue sites are in the bone (osteoblasts and chondroblasts), liver, and gastrointestinal tract. Other sites include the lung, spleen, placenta, kidney, and cells of the myeloid series. Within the cell it is associated with the Golgi apparatus and the endoplasmic reticulum. The phosphatase activity in serum can be separated into different isoenzymes. The predominant fraction seen in adult serum is derived from the liver, in contrast to a fraction of bone origin in the growing child and adolescent.

■ **If one cannot perform an ALP isoenzyme determination by electrophoresis, is there any other method of determining ALP source?**

Yes. Bone ALP can be distinguished from the hepatic isoenzyme by the fact that it is more rapidly inactivated at 55° C than liver ALP. Approximately half of the bone ALP activity can be eliminated within 8 minutes, whereas liver ALP requires an incubation period of approximately 20 minutes before half of its activity is eliminated.

■ **What are some of the inhibitors of ALP and which fractions do they affect?**

L-Phenylalanine inhibits intestinal phosphatase. L-Tryptophan and L-leucine inhibit placental phosphatase. L-Homoarginine, imidazole, and levamisole inhibit bone and liver phosphatase.[6]

■ **In what clinical situation may one see an elevated ALP level with no associated disease?**

In prepuberal children, ALP levels are uniformly elevated during the period of active bone growth, and increases in total nonspecific ALP may be seen. When a determination of isoenzymes is performed, it is found that both liver and bone fractions may be observed. In pregnancy, progressive elevation of ALP level is noted beginning at 15 weeks' gestation and progressing to term. Normal values are obtained between the third and sixth postpartum week.

■ **Are significant increases in ALP in adults ever normal?**

Excluding pregnant women, significant increases in ALP in an adult must be considered to be associated with disease until proven otherwise.

■ **Are there physiologic reasons for elevated ALP levels other than bone growth during infancy and adolescence?**

Yes. Bone healing following trauma and fracture of the skeletal system is associated with increased enzyme activity (stimulated osteoblasts). Surgical manipulation, such as insertion of an intramedullary rod, will also cause enzyme increases.

■ **Are isolated increases in ALP observed in infants always normal?**

No. Infants with intrahepatic biliary atresia (incomplete formation of the biliary system within the liver) may have marked increases in ALP activity.

■ **In what clinical situations may low serum ALP activity be noted unassociated with other enzyme changes?**

An inborn error of metabolism referred to as hypophosphatasia may be associated with low serum ALP activity. The cardinal features of this syndrome are an impaired mineralization of bone, reduced tissue and serum ALP activity, and the presence of phosphoethanolamine in the urine. These changes may be seen in infants, children, and adults. In adults there is usually a history of pathologic fractures and a childhood history of vitamin D–resistant rickets.

■ **What are the predominant causes of increased serum ALP associated with bone disease?**

Parathyroid hyperplasia, adenoma or carcinoma of the parathyroid, rickets, Paget's disease, metastatic carcinoma of the bone, and primary malignancy of the bone.

■ **What precautions should be taken when performing ALP determinations?**

Serum is the preferred specimen for ALP activity. Plasma is to be avoided because of the inhibitory effects of the anticoagulants.

■ **Are acid phosphatases as stable as ALP?**

Serum ALP is generally stable both at room temperature and at 4° C; however, acid phosphatase is very unstable.

■ **Of what value is determination of the immune precipitable ALP?**

It has been shown that a specific antibody directed against placental ALP can be used in immune precipitable techniques, and in such a situation, increases in this enzyme may be detected in significant amounts in some cases of malignancy. This enzyme is referred to by some as Regan enzyme.

■ **What may be the reason for some false increases in ALP?**

If the patient has received albumin derived from the human placenta, a marked elevation in ALP level may be noted.

■ **What is the character of the ALP isoenzymes?**

The liver isoenzyme is moderately heat labile, that of bone is extremely heat labile, and that of placental origin is heat stable. Additionally, the enzyme of placental origin is inhibited by phenylalanine.[6]

■ **Are there any discrepancies between acid phosphatase determinations on serum or on plasma?**

Yes. Acid phosphatase activity in serum is generally greater than that observed in plasma. This is probably caused by the liberation of the enzyme from platelets during the process of coagulation.

■ **Are isoenzymes of acid phosphatase clinically demonstrable?**

Yes. When different tissue extracts are separated on polyacrylamide gel, five isoenzyme bands are identifiable. Normal plasma contains only fraction 5. Serum on the other hand contains fractions 3 and 5. Fraction 3 is derived from the platelets consumed during the clotting process.[7]

■ **Is there normally a prostatic fraction present in serum?**

Prostatic acid phosphatase is not normally detectable in serum.

■ **What is characteristic of acid phosphatase arising from carcinoma of the prostate?**

Acid phosphatase arising from carcinoma of the prostate is formaldehyde stable, tartrate labile, and resistant to copper and can be inhibited by heparin. Additionally, 40% alcohol solution can inhibit prostatic acid phosphatase. Some authors have recommended the use of alpha-naphthol phosphate as a substrate in acid phosphatase determinations when the prostatic fraction is desired, because it is thought that alpha-naphthol phosphate is the most specific of all of the common substrates for prostatic acid phosphatase. It is good to be familiar with the type of substrate that one is using when performing an acid phosphatase determination and also to avoid the use of oxalate, heparin, and fluoride in tubes when drawing blood samples for acid phosphatase determination.

■ **What other clinical situations might cause an increase in acid phosphatase?**

Operative trauma, vigorous prostate massage, and infarcts (local tissue death) of the prostate are known to cause transient increases. Gaucher's disease is associated with striking increases in plasma acid phosphatase activity; disorders of platelets, particularly when destruction is excessive; liver disease, particularly cirrhosis; metastatic carcinoma of the liver; obstructive jaundice and hepatitis; bone disease, particularly in advanced Paget's disease and in cases of metastatic carcinoma; certain kidney diseases; hemolytic disease (because of the richness of acid phosphatase in the RBCs); and certain chromosomal abnormalities. In some instances, these increases can be best evaluated by performing the tests with and without inhibitors.

■ **What isoenzyme fractions are associated with carcinoma of the prostate?**

Fractions 2 and 4 are characteristically seen in association with carcinoma of the prostate.

■ **Which enzymes are useful in the evaluation of pancreatic disease?**

Amylase and lipase are the most useful.

■ **Are there any isoenzymes associated with amylase?**

Yes. Three bands have been observed on separation of serum and are presumably of pancreatic, salivary, and liver origin. Some believe that the liver supplies most of the amylase that is normally seen in the sera; however, in acute pancreatitis, total amylase increase in both serum and urine remains one of the single most important aids in confirming a diagnosis. Isoenzymes are less important.

■ **Is the diagnosis of pancreatitis usually based solely on the presence of observed enzyme activity?**

No. Frequently repeated determinations are required before a significant increase is seen. Also helpful in association with these determinations is serum calcium, which if low is supportive evidence of disease. It has been noted in critically ill patients with increased amylases that if serum calcium levels are not reduced but are normal or elevated, the possibility of hyperparathyroidism should be entertained.

■ **Are there any other factors involved in evaluating amylase increases?**

Yes. In the presence of renal disease, incomplete clearing of the serum amylase by the kidneys may inhibit the efficiency of the test.

■ **What is the significance of increases in serum amylase in patients with acute abdominal pain?**

Increases in serum amylase can be considered to be indicative of pancreatic disease. In one third of the cases, this may be accompanied by hypoglycemia. In general, amylase activity is inversely related to the severity of the pancreatic disease. Some authors believe that amylase values over 1,000 Somogyi units are consistent with surgically correctable lesions that frequently involve the biliary tract. Amylase activity between 200 and 500 units is associated with a majority of the patients with idiopathic pancreatitis and hemorrhagic pancreatitis.

■ **How soon can one expect an increase in amylase activity following abdominal pain?**

Within 2 to 12 hours of the onset of acute disease of the pancreas one may expect an increase in amylase activity, which will return to normal in healing patients by the fourth day.

■ **Does lipemia have any relationship to pancreatitis and amylase values?**

Yes. Significant lipemia is present in 3% to 12% of patients with pancreatitis. Of these patients, 75% will have normal amylase values.[8]

■ **Hyperamylasemia may be associated with both pancreatitis and common duct stone. Can the two conditions be differentiated?**

Yes, if one determines the amylase/creatinine clearance. Values of 8% or greater signify pancreatitis or pancreatitis with common duct stone; values of 3.5% or less signify common duct stone only. The normal value is 3.6% ± 0.2%. Use the following formula:

$$\frac{\text{Urinary amylase}}{\text{Serum amylase}} \times \frac{\text{Serum creatinine}}{\text{Urinary creatinine}} \times 100 = \% \text{ clearance}$$

It must be remembered that this data will be significantly altered if renal disease is present.[9-11]

■ **What other tests can be easily done in an effort to establish a differential diagnosis of acute abdominal pain?**

This depends somewhat on the age and sex of the patient. In a woman of childbearing age, a slide pregnancy test and a screening test for porphobilinogen are logical tests in addition to an amylase determination. This again depends on the clinical situation, and these tests could be coupled with total LD, isoenzyme, and CK determinations, the last two being helpful if cardiac or liver disease is responsible for the clinical symptoms. These tests do not exhaust the diagnostic possibilities as far as abdominal pain is concerned but generally are helpful.

■ **Are urinary amylases important?**

Determination of urinary amylase activity is preferred by some in suspected pancreatic disease principally because urinary amylase is more frequently increased, persists for a longer period of time, and reaches levels higher than those noted in the serum.

■ **Are isoenzymes of amylase of clinical importance?**

Yes. In patients with hyperamylasemia of unknown cause or in whom a response to therapy is atypical, isoenzyme determination may be helpful.

Salivary amylase and pancreatic amylase are readily separated on polyacrylamide gel. Salivary amylase has been reported to be associated with carcinoma of the lung and ovarian carcinomatosis. Pancreatic amylase is considered pathognomonic of abdominal disease.[12]

■ **What are some of the artifacts that may influence amylase activity?**

Opiates, hemolysis, storage of the serum sample at room temperature, and performing the amylase determination within the immediate postoperative period may cause spurious elevations of amylase level.

■ **What method is believed to be the best for true amylase activity?**

The saccharogenic method is best because this is the only method that truly demonstrates human isoamylase activity. By this technique, at least three different isoamylases have been noted, emanating from the pancreas, salivary gland, and liver. All three have an electrophoretic mobility similar to that of gamma globulin. The albumin activity is demonstrable only by amyloclastic technique, which is believed to be an artifact.

■ **How may a diagnosis of pancreatitis be ruled out by amylase activity?**

If the amylase level is not increased within the first 24 hours after the onset of symptoms, it is likely that the patient does not have acute pancreatitis.

■ **What other body fluids may be used to make a diagnosis of acute pancreatitis?**

Determination of amylase activity in peritoneal fluid has been found to be an advantage in the diagnosis of acute pancreatitis. Elevations of amylase level in the fluid are highly suggestive. Other conditions that may also be associated with elevation of peritoneal fluid amylase are a perforated small bowel and ectopic pregnancy.

■ **What is macroamylase?**

In macroamylasemia, the amylase is bound to an immunoglobulin, either IgA or IgG. This condition has been noted in association with malabsorption secondary to malignant lymphoma and villous atrophy. The amylase activity is elevated because this large molecule is not readily eliminated by the kidney as is the normal amylase. Because of this nonclearance by the kidney, concomitant elevations of amylase level are not noted in the urine.

■ **Of what value is the clinical interpretation of lipase?**

Lipases are present in fewer tissues than amylases, and for this reason increases are thought to be more specifically related to pancreatic disease. Inasmuch as serum lipase activity may persist up to a week longer than the serum amylase, a hyperlipasemia is regarded by some to be an invariable sign of acute pancreatic disease.

■ **What other conditions may be associated with increase in urinary lipase?**

Fat embolization of the lung has been noted to be the cause of increased release of lipase from the injured lung tissue.

■ **Does serum lipase activity correlate with severity of pancreatic disease?**

Good correlation does not usually exist, because lipase activity tends to lag behind the increase in serum amylase by approximately 24 hours. The magnitude of increase, however, does tend to parallel that of the amylase. Additionally, abnormal lipase activity can be detected for up to 14 days after the initial onset of acute pancreatitis.

■ **Does mumps cause an elevation of serum lipase activity?**

No.

■ **Which enzymes are most likely to be affected physiologically by a normal pregnancy?**

Increase in ALP may be normally noted during pregnancy. This is principally related to the placental fraction. Additionally, slow but continual rise in CK of from 3 to 5 times the normal value has been observed in the third trimester, particularly at the time of delivery.

■ **What effects do oral contraceptives have on enzymes?**

Elevations of ALT level have been found to be a sensitive indicator of apparent liver dysfunction when increased sensitivity to the pill occurs. This increase in ALT may be as much as 2 times that of AST. Peak incidence for increased enzymes is observed during the second month. The return to normal has been observed within 4 weeks after the drug has been discontinued. This further points out the value of screening patients before administration of the pill.

■ **Does toxemia in pregnancy affect enzymes?**

ALP may be increased. Additionally, acid phosphatase increases are noted. In the preeclamptic states, the values may be 2 times the nonpregnant level and greater than 65% of that normally seen during the third trimester.

■ **What is the value of performing a ceruloplasmin determination?**

Ceruloplasmin is a copper oxidase that occurs in plasma. Increases have been noted in association with oral contraceptives and pregnancy; however, its principle clinical use is in diagnosis of Wilson's disease, in which a marked decrease in activity is observed. Other causes for increases are Hodgkin's disease, hyperthyroidism, and acute inflammatory states.

■ **How many cholinesterases exist?**

Two major cholinesterases exist: true, or type 1, which is acetylcholinesterase, and pseudo-, or type 2, cholinesterase.

■ **Where is acetylcholinesterase located?**

Acetylcholinesterase is found in erythrocytes and in nerve tissue, particularly at the point of synapse. Pseudocholinesterase is present in the serum.

■ **What is the clinical usefulness of cholinesterase determination?**

A decrease in serum cholinesterase (type 2) is associated with hepatitis, cirrhosis, and carcinoma of the liver. Measurement of the serum erythrocyte cholinesterase (type 1) is valuable in the determination of exposure to organic phosphate insecticides. In such a situation, activity may be reduced up to 40%.

■ **Of what further importance is the determination of pseudocholinesterase (type 2)?**

Certain individuals have a genetically altered cholinesterase, referred to as an atypical variant, that cannot hydrolyze succinylcholine. This atypical enzyme may be distinguished from normal pseudocholinesterase because it is not inhibited by either fluoride or dibucaine. Ten possible genetic combinations exist; however, those patients who have a homozygous abnormality will have a low dibucaine number and a low fluoride number.

■ **Where is aldolase located?**

Aldolase is located principally in the skeletal muscle and in lesser amounts in the heart, liver, and red cells.

■ **In what clinical conditions are increases in aldolase observed?**

Increases are primarily observed in muscle disease such as muscular dystrophy and polymyositis; they may also be observed in liver disease and myocardial infarction.

■ **What are two general classes of hormones?**

Hormones are classified as steroid and nonsteroid. The latter can be subdivided into peptide and nonpeptide. The peptide group of pituitary origin includes polypeptides, proteins, and glycoproteins. The nonpituitary peptides include insulin, glucagon, and gastrin. The nonpeptides include aromatic amines such as thyroxine, catechols, and histamine. All of these hormones exert their effect on tissues distant to the site of hormone production. (NOTE: This discussion does not include the tissue hormones, such as kinins and prostaglandins, which exert their effect at the site of their production.)

■ **What are examples of pituitary peptide hormones?**

1. Polypeptide (mol. wt. 2,000 to 4,000 daltons): adrenocorticotropic hormone (ACTH) and melanocyte-stimulating hormone (MSH).

2. Protein (mol. wt. approximately 22,000): growth hormone and prolactin.

3. Glycoprotein (mol. wt. 26,000 to 40,000): thyroid-stimulating hormone (TSH), follicle-stimulating hormone (FSH), and luteinizing hormone (LH). Human chorionic gonadotropin (HCG) is also a glycoprotein but is not of pituitary origin.

(NOTE: The releasing hormones, such as thyrotropin-releasing hormone [TRH], are also peptides, but they are of very small molecular weight and originate in the hypothalamus.)

■ **Distinguish the pituitary hormones and the steroid hormones on the basis of their different modes of action.**

The pituitary hormones are of a larger molecular weight than steroid hormones and consequently do not enter the cell. Rather, they bind with specific receptors on the effector cell and activate adenylcyclase. The latter is a membrane-bound enzyme that converts adenosine triphosphate (ATP) to cyclic adenosine 3'5' monophosphate (AMP), which in turn causes the cell to act in a specific manner.

In contrast, steroids have a very small molecular weight. They enter the cell and combine with cytoplasmic receptors within the cell. The hormone is then transported to the nucleus of the cell, causing the generation of a messenger RNA. The messenger RNA exits the nucleus, returns to the cytoplasm, and stimulates the ribosomes to generate specific proteins.[13]

■ **What is cyclic AMP?**

Cyclic AMP is the product of the interaction between a peptide hormone and a membrane-bound enzyme, adenylcyclase, located in the effector cell. The activation of the enzyme transforms ATP to cyclic AMP. The latter carries out the work of the hormone within the cell, i.e., affecting the specific activities of the cell.[14]

■ **What is meant by first messenger, second messenger, and third messenger when speaking of peptide hormone action?**

First messenger refers to the hormone itself. Second messenger refers to cyclic AMP. Third messenger refers to the specific action carried out by the cell, e.g., gluconeogenesis, steroidogenesis.[15]

■ **How are hormones controlled?**

Hormones are controlled by biofeedback mechanisms and some also by enzymatic degradation.[16]

■ **Are there special features of the glycoprotein class that have special laboratory significance?**

Yes. These hormones consist of two subunits, alpha and beta. The alpha subunit is identical in all glycoprotein hormones in all species. Beta subunits are different in each species (i.e., species-specific) and confer immunospecificity on their component hormone. The beta subunits, however, have no biologic activity unless coupled with the alpha subunit.

■ **Can beta subunits be measured?**

Yes. Routine tests for beta subunits of HCG are currently used to aid in the diagnosis of normal pregnancy and molar pregnancy. The latter can be distinguished from the former by measurement of LH. In a normal pregnancy, both values will be elevated early; in a molar pregnancy, the HCG level will be elevated and LH level will be low.

■ **Can tumors produce alpha and beta subunits of HCG?**

Yes. Carcinoma of the testis, liver, gastrointestinal tract, hematopoietic system, breast, and pancreas have been reported to produce alpha and/or beta subunits of HCG.[17-18]

■ **What are releasing hormones?**

Releasing hormones are very small peptides secreted by "peptidergic," or peptide-producing, neurons in the hypothalamus. These hormones act on the pituitary gland, causing a release of specific tropic hormones from the anterior pituitary; e.g., TRH stimulates the elaboration of TSH from the pituitary.[19]

■ **What are other examples of releasing hormones?**

Other releasing hormones are corticotropin-releasing hormone (CRH), which is responsible for the release of ACTH, luteinizing hormone–releasing hormone (LH-RH), and growth hormone–releasing hormone (GH-RH). Also, inhibitory hormones are produced by the hypothalamus, such as prolactin-inhibiting hormone and growth hormone–inhibiting hormone. The latter is also called somatotropin release–inhibiting factor (SRIF) or, more commonly, somatostatin.

■ **Why are releasing and inhibiting hormones important?**

Ultimately it may turn out that each hormone produced by the anterior pituitary gland is under the dual control of a releasing hormone and an inhibiting hormone. Thus, the overall effects of the feedback mechanisms that control pituitary function are mediated not only by direct effect on the pituitary but also via the specialized hormones of the hypothalamus.

Furthermore, it can be seen that any end-organ dysfunction (thyroid, adrenal, etc.) may be related not only to primary failure of that organ but also to failure of the pituitary to produce the appropriate tropic hormones or to failure of the hypothalamus to elaborate the appropriate releasing hormone.

■ **What is somatostatin?**

Somatostatin (or SRIF) is a tetradecapeptide derived from the hypothalamus that inhibits secretion of immunoreactive growth hormone. It also inhibits thyrotropin secretion induced by TRH. However, it does not affect prolactin release, which is also stimulated by TRH.[20]

■ **Does somatostatin affect any endocrine activity other than that of the pituitary?**

Yes. Somatostatin inhibits insulin secretion and lowers glucose levels in normal subjects.

■ **Can somatostatin aid in the treatment of diabetic ketoacidosis?**

Yes. Somatostatin reduces alpha-cell secretion from pancreatic islets, and as a result, glucagon secretion is suppressed. For this reason somatostatin is used as an adjunct to insulin in management of diabetes.

■ **Which tests are best to evaluate growth hormone, i.e., determination of impaired growth hormone release?**

Levodopa and insulin-induced hypoglycemia are equally effective as stimulus to growth hormone release. Levodopa has an advantage in that is can be given orally. However, insulin-induced hypoglycemia is still the most popular test.[21]

■ **What is the basic structure of a steroid?**

The basic structure of a steroid is a 17-carbon aromatic compound referred to as cyclopentanophenanthrene. To this 17-carbon molecule are added the two angular groups at positions 10 and 13. The angular carbon at position 13 is carbon-18, and the angular carbon added at position 10 is carbon-19. Those carbons added at position 17 are carbon-20 and carbon-21.

■ **What are the androgenic compounds?**

The androgenic compounds are the C-19 compounds. These include the steroids, which have two angular methyl groups, one at C-10 and the other at C-13, and which have at position 17 either a keto or hydroxyl group rather than additional carbons.

■ **What are the estrogenic compounds?**

The estrogenic compounds are C-18 compounds, which only have one additional methyl group at position 13. Additionally, aromatization of the first ring is characteristic of estrogen, that is, the first ring, or A-ring, is converted into a benzene configuration.

■ **What are the progestational compounds?**

Progestational compounds are C-21 compounds that are similar to the adrenocortical hormones but have a methyl group rather than a hydroxyl group at position 21, which is characteristic of the adrenocorticoids.

■ **What are the structural requirements for activity by the adrenocortical hormones?**

The requirements are a double bond between positions 4 and 5, a ketone group in position 3, and a ketone group in position 20.

■ **Which radicals impart a specific activity to the adrenocorticoids?**

C-21 hydroxylation enhances sodium retention and is effective in carbohydrate metabolism. C-17 hydroxylated compounds increase carbohydrate activity. This includes hydrocortisone and cortisone. C-11 oxygenated compounds decrease sodium retention and are also necessary for carbohydrate activity. This group includes corticosterone and dehydrocorticosterone. They inhibit membrane permeability and have a role in suppressing lymphocytes, eosinophils, and basophils. C-11 deoxygenated compounds (no oxygen) have a profound effect on water and electrolyte metabolism. This group of compounds includes aldosterone.

■ **Summarize the total effect of adrenocortical compounds.**

The adrenocortical compounds have an effect on glucose metabolism, causing gluconeogenesis and hyperglycemia. For this reason, they are thought to be diabetogenic. Because of their effect on acid mucopolysaccharides and chondroitin sulfate, adrenocortical compounds lead to osteoporosis. The corticoids induce negative nitrogen balance and thus are considered catabolic. They tend to promote release of unesterified fatty acids from adipose tissue and are therefore lipemic. They induce lysis of lymph nodes, causing lymphopenia, and therefore are considered to be immunosuppressive. Additionally, they are anti-inflammatory and have a profound effect on sodium and potassium metabolism.

■ **What is considered to be the common precursor of all steroids?**

Cholesterol is the common precursor of all steroids.

■ **What are the sources of the steroids that are generally determined in the clinical lab?**

Sources of steroids are adrenocorticoids from the adrenal glands, androgens from the testes, and estrogens from the ovaries.

■ **What is the major human glucocorticoid and how can it be determined?**

Cortisol. This steroid can now be assayed by radioimmunoassay.[22]

■ **Are estrogen and androgen produced only by the ovary and testis, respectively?**

No. Although estrogens are produced predominantly by the ovary, small amounts are produced by the adrenal gland. Conversely, the androgens are produced predominantly by the testis; however, one third to one quarter of the androgens are produced by the adrenal gland in the form of ketosteroids.

■ **What are 17-ketosteroids?**

The 17-ketosteroids are that group of compounds having a ketone group at position 17 of the D-ring.

■ **What is the Zimmermann reaction?**

The Zimmermann reaction is the reaction used in the clinical laboratory for determining the level of the 17-ketosteroids.

■ **What is the principal reagent in the Zimmermann reaction?**

The principal reagent is dinitrobenzene in association with methanol and potassium hydroxide.

■ **What is the purpose of the Zimmermann reaction?**

The Zimmermann reaction reflects the amount of adrenal and testicular activity. In the male, two thirds to three fourths of the 17-ketosteroids are derived from the testes and one third to one quarter from the adrenal. In the normal female, the majority of 17-ketosteroids arise from the adrenal; however, some small amount may arise from the hilar region of the ovary.

■ **What does the Zimmermann reaction measure?**

The Zimmermann reaction measures 17-ketosteroids arising from the adrenal, principally dehydroepiandrosterone and 11-ketoetiocholanolone, and from the testes, principally androsterone and etiocholanolone. The test does *not* measure testosterone, which is not a 17-ketosteroid but an androgen that has a hydroxyl group at position 17.

■ **What is the clinical significance of increases in the 17-ketosteroids?**

Increases are noted in adrenocortical carcinoma (particularly in the form of increased dehydroepiandrosterone), in acromegaly, in tumors of the testis, and in masculinizing tumors of the ovary. Decreases are noted in Addison's disease, panhypopituitarism, myxedema, and nephrosis.

■ **What are the Porter-Silber chromogens?**

The Porter-Silber chromogens are the 17-hydroxycorticoids that combine with phenylhydrazine. The phenylhydrazine reacts with the ketone group present at position 20, forming a chromogen when a hydroxyl group is present at positions 17 and 21.

■ **What does the 17-hydroxycorticoid determination measure?**

The 17-hydroxycorticoid determination principally measures biologically active cortisone, hydrocortisone, and 11-deoxycortisol. Measurement of the corticoids is generally considered to be a better indication of adrenocortical function than measurement of the 17-ketosteroids.

■ **In what clinical situations are there increases in 17-hydroxycorticoids?**

Cushing's syndrome, eclampsia, and acute pancreatitis manifest such increases.

■ **In what clinical situations are measures of hydroxycorticoids low?**

In Addison's disease and hypopituitarism the measures are low.

■ **What are the 17-ketogenics?**

The 17-ketogenics include the 17-hydroxycorticoids and those compounds having hydroxyl groups on positions 17, 20, and 21, as well as those having a hydroxyl group only on position 17 and the ketone group on position 20 with a methyl group at position 21. These compounds include cortisone, hydrocortisone, 17-hydroxyprogesterone, pregnanetriol, and the tetrahydro derivatives of cortisone, cortisol, and cortexolone.

■ **What is the reaction whereby the 17-ketogenics are determined?**

First is a reduction phase incorporating the use of sodium borohydride, followed by an oxidative phase using sodium bismuthate or periodate, forming a 17-keto group. Subsequently a standard Zimmermann reaction is employed using dinitrobenzene.

■ **What are the clinical conditions associated with an increase in 17-ketogenics?**

The ketogenics are sensitive in the evaluation of adrenocortical activity and are particularly useful in the diagnosis of the adrenogenital syndrome.

■ **What are the major enzymatic steps in the formation of steroids from cholesterol?**

First, the cholesterol is enzymatically converted to progesterone. From that point, two major sequential pathways of enzymatic alterations of the molecule occur. The first is the hydroxylation of the C-17, forming hydroxyprogesterone, followed by the hydroxylation of the C-21, forming 17-hydroxyprogesterone, and finally the hydroxylation of the C-11 position, forming cortisol. Cortisol is then converted to cortisone. By other pathways, 17-hydroxyprogesterone can form both deoxycorticosterone, corticosterone, and aldosterone, which are the principal sodium- and potassium-controlling substances. Second, progesterone can go on to form androstenedione and testosterone, which in turn form the estrogens.

■ **What is the principal stimulator of the adrenal gland?**

ACTH stimulates the adrenal gland.

■ **What is the principal feedback substance produced by the adrenal gland that tends to turn ACTH off?**

Cortisol is the principal feedback substance.

■ **What happens clinically when cortisol is not produced or is produced in low quantities?**

Unopposed stimulation of the adrenal gland by ACTH occurs, causing hyperplasia of the gland and elaboration of the alternate pathway metabolites.

■ **Which metabolites occur chiefly in the urine?**

The metabolites that occur in the urine are present in four forms: (1) the biologically active form of the hormones; (2) the biologically inactive form of the hormone, principally tetrahydrocorticosterone and tetrahydrocortisone; (3) 17-ketosteroids, which are mainly conjugated; and (4) a small amount of pregnanediol and pregnanetriol. Aldosterone is also elaborated in the urine, usually in the inactive form; however, some free and conjugated aldosterone is also excreted.

■ **What are the principal 17-ketosteroids found in the urine?**

Two forms of the 17-ketosteroids are excreted in the urine: the alpha ketosteroid (androsterone) and etiocholanolone. Both of these substances are soluble in digitonin. The beta 17-ketosteroids, which include epiandrosterone and dihydroepiandrosterone, are precipitated by digitonin.

■ **What is the effect of dexamethasone on the Porter-Silber chromogens?**

The Porter-Silber compounds are predominantly cortisol and cortisone. Inasmuch as dexamethasone has an inhibitory effect on ACTH production, the result is a suppression of the principal 17-hydroxycorticoid, cortisol.

■ **Of what clinical use is the dexamethasone suppression test?**

This test distinguishes between primary and secondary adrenal hyperplasia.

■ **What is the effect of metyrapone on steroid metabolism?**

Metyrapone (Metopirone) is a selective inhibitor of 11-hydroxylation. Therefore, this substance prevents the formation of cortisol, and an accumulation of cortisol precursors is measured as 17-hydroxycorticoids in the urine. Without the formation of cortisol, the feedback mechanism for shutting off ACTH production is ineffective. Therefore, in a normal individual, metyrapone causes an increased stimulation of adrenal activity by causing more ACTH production. This is manifested by an increase in total ketogenic steroids, a suppression of cortisol, and an increase in cortisol precursors.

■ **How is the metyrapone test used clinically?**

In cases of adrenal hyperplasia, metyrapone will cause a twofold increase in urinary 17-hydroxycorticoids. In carcinoma of the adrenal gland, no change will occur.

■ **What is the effect of dexamethasone on the urinary excretion of 17-hydroxycorticoids?**

In the normal individual, dexamethasone suppresses ACTH; therefore, the urinary 17-hydroxycorticoids are decreased. In cases of hyperplasia of the adrenal gland caused by increased stimulation by the pituitary, the preadministration values for 17-hydroxycorticoids are elevated and no suppression occurs after administration of low doses of dexamethasone. However, if the dose is increased, effective suppression of hyperplastic glands occurs. This is in contrast to primary tumors of the adrenal gland, which elaborate their own cortisol and thus have already suppressed pituitary ACTH. In that instance, the administration of dexamethasone has no effect.

■ **What is characteristic of the normal physiologic elaboration of 17-hydroxycorticoids?**

A diurnal variation in the elaboration of 17-hydroxycorticoids occurs. A level of approximately 20μg/dl appears at 6 AM, falling to approximately half of the morning sample by 6 PM of the same day, only to return to the higher fasting level by 6 AM the following day. Characteristically, loss of the diural variation of the level of plasma 17-hydroxycorticoids is indicative of Cushing's syndrome.

■ **What are the four major manifestations of hyperfunction of the adrenal gland?**

The four major manifestations are (1) increased secretion of all of the adrenocortical hormones, as observed in Cushing's syndrome; (2) hypersecretion of androgens, as seen in the adrenogenital syndrome; (3) exclusive hypersecretion of estrogen, as seen in the feminizing syndrome that occurs in males; (4) exclusive hypersecretion of aldosterone, as observed in primary hyperaldosteronism.

■ **What are the common causes of hyperfunctioning of the adrenal gland?**

The causes of such hyperfunction are (1) pituitary tumor causing hyperplasia of the adrenal gland, (2) primary hyperplasia of the adrenal gland, and (3) tumors occurring primarily in the adrenal gland. Certain nonendocrine tumors may also produce an ACTHlike substance, e.g., oat-cell carcinoma of the lung.

■ **What are the significant laboratory tests for diagnosing adrenocortical hyperfunction?**

Significant laboratory tests and results include the following: increase in 17-hydroxy compounds, principally cortisone, increase in 17-ketosteroids, usually increase in the 17-ketogenics, and loss of the diurnal variation in blood cortisol secretion.

■ **What tests are used to distinguish between pituitary tumor, primary adrenal hyperplasia, and tumor of the adrenal gland?**

The suppression tests, principally the dexamethasone suppression test and the metyrapone suppression test, are used.

■ **What are the principal causes of hypofunctioning of the adrenal gland (Addison's disease)?**

The principal causes of such hypofunction are (1) atrophy of the adrenocortex (55% of cases), (2) tuberculosis (approximately 40% of cases), and (3) other causes, including metastatic carcinoma, trauma, and histoplasmosis (approximately 5% of cases).

■ **Which tests are most likely to be affected by a hypofunctioning adrenal gland?**

Decreased 17-ketosteroids, decreased 17-hydroxycorticoids, and inadequate increases in 17-hydroxycorticoids after ACTH stimulation will most likely result from such hypofunction.

■ **What controls the function of the anterior pituitary gland?**

The anterior pituitary gland is controlled by regulating hormones known as releasing hormones and inhibiting hormones that are produced by the hypothalamus.

■ **Which releasing hormones have been identified?**

Releasing hormone for ACTH, thyrotropin, LH, and FSH as well as several others have been isolated.

■ **Have isolated deficiencies in the production of the releasing hormones been described?**

Yes.

■ **How may a diagnosis of hyperfunctioning of the pituitary gland be made on a laboratory basis?**

In the past the determination of hormones elaborated by the pituitary gland was tedious because these tests involved bioassay techniques. Radioimmunoassay procedures for FSH, LH, thyrotropic hormone, growth hormone, and prolactin are currently available. ACTH may also be determined by a radioimmunoassay procedure.

■ **What are some of the common causes for pituitary anterior lobe deficiency?**

The most common causes are pituitary infarction in women following pregnancy, destruction of the pituitary by tumor, granuloma, and trauma. The tumors most commonly associated with pituitary deficiencies are chromophobe adenomas and cranial pharyngiomas.

■ **In primary hypopituitarism, what is the usual sequence of end-organ failure?**

The signs, symptoms, and physical and laboratory findings are consistent with sequential failure of production of growth hormone, gonadotropin, TSH, and ACTH, i.e., successive failure of growth (in a child), gonads, thyroid, and adrenal cortex.

■ **What is antidiuretic hormone (ADH) and how does it work?**

ADH is an octapeptide made in the supraoptic and paraventricular nuclei of the brain. It plays a major role in the body's regulation of water by acting on the distal tubules of the kidney, where specific receptors are located. The structure of the membrane is altered by cyclic AMP changing the diffusion characteristics of the cell and thus allowing water and certain solutes to be reabsorbed.

■ **What is the function of the posterior lobe of the pituitary gland with respect to ADH?**

The posterior lobe of the pituitary gland is composed of the axons of cells arising in the hypothalamus. Osmoreceptors are also located in the hypothalamus and respond to changes in blood osmolality. When osmolality levels are high, the cell nucleus in the hypothalamus is stimulated, releasing the hormone from the axonal portion of the cell in the posterior lobe of the pituitary gland.

■ **What disease is associated with faulty production of ADH?**

Diabetes insipidus is associated with faulty production of ADH. The causes of this abnormality include tumor, inflammation, granuloma, trauma, and vascular thrombosis.

■ **What tests are clinically employed to diagnose diabetes insipidus?**

The urinary output is measured under constant water-loading conditions and using hypertonic saline solution, nicotine, and vasopressin. If lack of response to these agents is noted, a diagnosis of diabetes insipidus is indicated. However, certain inappropriate responses in ADH production are noted to be associated particularly with hypovolemia following bleeding, edematous states (as noted in cardiac failure), nephrotic syndrome, and cirrhosis. Additionally, certain malignant tumors, particularly of the lung, are associated with inappropriate ADH release.

■ **What are the laboratory manifestations of primary hyperaldosteronism?**

Low serum potassium level associated with excessive urinary loss of both potassium and hydrogen ions (hypokalemic alkalosis) is accompanied by an increased serum sodium level and increased water reabsorption. This results in hypernatremia and hypervolemia, usually without manifestation of edema.

■ **Which two clinical tests most characterize primary hyperaldosteronism?**

The two tests are (1) increased urinary excretion of aldosterone, and (2) depressed elaboration of plasma renin.

■ **How is the hypertension associated with hyperaldosteronism differentiated from the hypertension caused by renal vascular disease (secondary hyperaldosteronism)?**

In renal vascular disease, renin (an enzyme elaborated by the kidney that converts angiotensinogen to angiotensin 1) is increased, whereas in primary hyperaldosteronism, renin activity is very low.

■ **What is Bartter's syndrome?**

Bartter's syndrome is characterized by high aldosterone level, high plasma renin activity, and normal blood pressure.

■ **What are the characteristics of infantile adrenogenital syndrome?**

In infantile adrenogenital syndrome, simple virilism is caused by faulty biosynthesis of the adrenocorticosteroids. This results principally from an enzymatic block in hydroxylation of the cortisol precursors. With a deficiency of cortisol and unopposed elaboration of ACTH, adrenal hyperplasia occurs and is predominantly manifested by masculinization of the external genitalia of female infants.

■ **What is the most common enzymatic block responsible for infantile adrenogenital syndrome?**

The block of 21-hydroxylation is the most common.

■ **Is the adrenogenital syndrome noted in adults?**

Yes. The cause of adrenogenital syndrome in adults may also be selective enzymatic blocks in production of cortisol; however, it may be associated with adenomas or carcinoma. When it occurs in a female, evidence of excessive 17-ketosteroid production is noted associated with clinical evidence of masculinization. The urinary 17-ketosteroids are only moderately increased in hyperplasias of a benign order but may be markedly increased in cases of adenoma and adenocarcinoma.

■ **What is the function of the adrenal medulla?**

The medullary portion of the adrenal gland produces substances that are responsible for the clinical signs of fight or flight, i.e., sweating, rapid pulse rate, increase of blood pressure, flushed face, dilated pupils, and loss of visceral function.

■ **What are the principal substances found in the urine that emanate from the adrenal medulla?**

Epinephrine, norepinephrine, metanephrine, normetanephrine, and vanillylmandelic acid are found in urine.

■ **What are the principal metabolites of the adrenal medulla found in the urine?**

The composition is the following: (1) free vanillylmandelic acid, approximately 40%; (2) conjugated and free metanephrine associated with conjugated and free normetanephrine, 40%; and (3) the combined catecholamines, epinephrine, and norepinephrine, the remaining 20%. The ratio of epinephrine to norepinephrine is approximately 1:4.

■ **What is the clinical significance of increases in these catecholamines?**

In association with a tumor of the adrenal medulla (referred to as pheochromocytoma), increases in the catecholamines occur. Those tumors arising from the adrenal gland proper tend to secrete norepinephrine and epinephrine, whereas those tumors arising outside of the adrenal tend predominantly to produce norepinephrine.

■ **Should any precautions be taken before a laboratory evaluation of the elaboration of vanillylmandelic acid is performed?**

Yes. The patient should avoid coffee, tea, chocolate, bananas, vanilla extracts, and drugs such as glyceryl guaiacolate, aminosalicylic acid, chlorpromazine, and bronchodilators.

■ **What is the function of the thyroid gland?**

The thyroid gland synthesizes, stores, and secretes thyroid hormone under stimulation by the pituitary gland.

■ **What is the basic physiology involved in thyroid hormone synthesis?**

Inorganic iodide is absorbed by the gastrointestinal tract and circulates as iodide either to be trapped by the thyroid gland or to be excreted via the salivary gland or urinary tract. The thyrotropic hormone emanating from the pituitary gland enhances the trapping of iodide by the gland, whereas substances such as thiocyanate can block this activity. In the thyroid cells, the iodide is converted by an oxidative enzyme into iodine. This activity can be blocked by thiouracil. The oxidized iodine is then rapidly used in the iodination of tyrosine to form mono- and diiodotyrosine. Sulfonamide derivatives interfere with the iodination of tyrosine. The combination of the mono- and diiodinated tyrosine results in the formation of thyroxine (T4) and triiodothyronine (T3). These substances are then stored in the gland in a large molecular form known as thyroglobulin.

■ **How are the thyroid hormones released from the thyroid gland?**

When the thyroid gland is stimulated by TSH, the hormones T4 and T3 are released from thyroglobulin by proteolytic enzymes.

■ **What happens to the released hormones?**

The released hormones (mostly T4) travel to the peripheral tissues in both free and combined forms. The major portion, however, is combined with the thyroid-binding globulin (TBG) in the serum. In the peripheral tissues, T4 is converted to T3. Approximately 80% of the circulating T3 is derived in this manner.

■ **Where is the major thyroxine-binding protein located?**

The binding protein is located between the alpha-1 and alpha-2 globulins; this globulin is known as an interalpha globulin.

■ **Which of the hormones is the most biologically active?**

Although T4 is present in larger amounts in the serum, T3 is the most active of the two.

■ **What is the value of determining TBG?**

TBG is determined to differentiate between abnormal T4 levels due to glandular dysfunction and those due to binding protein. Some methods make allowances for fluctuations in TBG, namely, determination of the effective thyroid ratio (ETR).

■ **What is reverse T3 (rT3)?**

Reverse T3 (3,3'5' triiodothyronine) is an inactive product of peripheral T4 metabolism. T4 is monodeiodinated in two ways, resulting in the formation of T3 (3,3'5' triiodothyronine) and rT3. Most of the T4 is normally converted to the active T3 form.

■ **Is the peripheral conversion of T4 ever such that the production of rT3 is favored?**

Yes. Infection, cirrhosis, severe malnutrition, and dexamethasone therapy result in increased rT3 production. The level of rT3 is also markedly elevated in newborns. The exact mechanism, however, is not well understood.[23-24]

■ **What is the feedback to the pituitary gland that inhibits TSH production?**

T4 is the principal substance that inhibits the release of TSH.

■ **Can globulins other than the interalpha globulin bind the thyroid hormones?**

Yes. Thyroxine can also bind to prealbumin and, to a lesser degree, to albumin. Triiodothyronine can bind to albumin; however, it does not bind to prealbumin.

■ **What are the clinical laboratory manifestations of hyperthyroidism?**

The manifestations are increase in T4, increase in T3, a normal or low cholesterol level, decrease in phospholipids, and a low uric acid level. There may be an increase in blood sugar, which can produce a diabetic tolerance curve, and there may be a relative lymphocytosis.

■ **Is the determination of TSH valuable in diagnosing hyperthyroidism?**

Not usually. It is generally accepted that the TSH level should be low; however, the test is more significant when making a diagnosis of hypothyroidism.

■ **Are there substances that can interefere with the thyroid test?**

Interference on thyroid tests depends on the methods employed. If the competitive binding analysis for serum thyroxine is performed, there is little or no interference by inorganic or organic iodides. This problem is present when tests of thyroid activity are performed using direct chemical measurements.

■ **Does an elevated or low value of serum total thyroxine always mean increased or decreased production of thyroid hormone?**

No. Alteration in the level of TBG will alter the value of serum T4. If a serum free-thyroxine test is performed (FT4), variations in TBG will not affect the final result.

■ **Can the binding capacity of TBG and thyroid-binding prealbumin be altered?**

Yes. Estrogens and estrogen-containing oral contraceptives can cause increases in TBG. Conversely, salicylates and phenytoin (Dilantin) tend to displace the hormone from the globulin by competition.

■ **What is the effect on the T3-by-column caused by alterations in TBG?**

T3 uptake varies inversely to the amount of thyroid-binding protein available. When there is an increase in binding protein, as seen in pregnancy, the T3 values will be lower. When the protein levels are low, the T3 values will be elevated.

■ **What laboratory test of thyroid function circumvents the effect of protein alteration?**

The determination of free thyroxine circumvents the effects of altered protein concentration.

■ **Is the determination of ^{131}I uptake by the thyroid an effective test?**

Uptake of the ^{131}I tracer continues to be helpful in distinguishing thyroid hyperfunction from normal function; however, it is inadequate to distinguish euthyroid states from hypothyroid states. It is also useful in the diagnosis of thyroiditis.

■ **By what method may TSH be evaluated?**

The determination of TSH by radioimmunoassay is the most sensitive method. It is used to distingish between primary hypothyroidism caused by primary thyroid failure and secondary hypothyroidism caused by pituitary failure. The serum TSH level is elevated in the former and low or absent in the latter.

■ **How can one best evaluate hypothalamic hypothyroidism?**

This can best be done by affirming thyrotropin (TSH) deficiency. A direct measurement of TRH by radioimmunoassay will confirm an associated deficiency of TSH.[25]

■ **What is LATS?**

LATS stands for long-acting thyroid stimulator. It is an immunoglobulin produced by lymphocytes and is found in the serum of patients with Graves' disease.

■ **What tests are useful in monitoring a patient who is receiving replacement therapy for a hypofunctioning thyroid gland?**

There is evidence to suggest that T4 is converted peripherally to T3. Consequently, methods for T4 determination are inadequate, because circulating T3 is not measured by the usual techniques of measuring T4. Therefore, the patient may be euthyroid (normal) while taking T3 and still have a low serum total T4 and free T4 level. Generally, patients who frequently take desiccated thyroid have a low normal or slightly decreased serum total T4 level, whereas patients taking a mixture of T3 and T4 have a serum total T4 level within the normal range. Some believe that the best guide is the determination of serum TSH level, which will be in the normal range if the patient is receiving adequate therapy and elevated if not.

■ **What is T3 toxicosis?**

T3 toxicosis, a variant of Graves' disease, is characterized by a normal or low serum T4 level, an elevated T3 level, and a normal TBG level. This is associated with elevated or normal ^{131}I uptake by the thyroid gland, which cannot be suppressed when T3 is administered.

■ **What is calcitonin?**

Calcitonin is a polypeptide produced by the parafollicular cells of the thyroid, which cause hypocalcemia. Similar cells are observed in the thymus and parathyroid gland.

■ **What is the effect of calcitonin on the human body?**

Calcitonin decreases bone resorption, increases urinary excretion of calcium and phosphorus, and induces hypocalcemia and hypophosphatemia.

■ **In what situation is there an increase in calcitonin?**

In medullary carcinoma of the thyroid, increases in calcitonin are known, and there may be associated hyperparathyroidism, multiple tumors of the adrenal medulla (pheochromocytoma), and tumors of the mucous membrane (ganglioneuroma).

■ **What is myxedema?**

Myxedema is a disease caused by hypofunctioning of the thyroid gland. It is characterized by low T4 level, low T3 level, low ^{131}I uptake, elevated cholesterol level, low 17-ketosteroid level, and low basal metabolic rate.

■ **What are the causes of myxedema?**

Myxedema may be caused primarily by failure of the thyroid to produce hormones, or it may be secondary to pituitary hypofunctioning.

■ **How can one distinguish between primary myxedema and secondary myxedema?**

In primary myxedema, TSH values are high and values for T3 and T4 cannot be elevated by administration of additional TSH. In secondary myxedema, T3 and T4 levels may be elevated after the administration of TSH.

■ **Can hypothyroidism occur in infants?**

Yes. Cretinism is the result of congenital absence of the thyroid hormone, or it may be associated with nonfunctioning goiters or goiters incapable of synthesizing normal hormones.

■ **What is the functional status of the thyroid gland in the newborn and what changes take place within the first 24 hours?**

The newborn is initially T3 deficient, apparently because of decreased peripheral conversion of T4 and T3. Soon after birth, a rapid rise in TSH occurs and is believed to cause an increase in the thyroid secretion of T3. At 24 hours, the newborn total T4 reaches a level of $16\mu g/dl$, with total T3 reaching a level of 419 ng/dl.

The level of rT3 in cord blood, however, is 151 ng/dl as compared with 40 ng/dl in adults. These elevated values of rT3 will return to normal adult values by 10 days.[24,26]

■ **Is screening of newborns for hypothyroidism important?**

Yes. Approximately 1 in 6,000 infants are born with hypothyroidism.[27]

■ **What methods are used to effect this screening?**

Measurements of T4 and TSH are used by some. However, others have proposed measuring diiodothyronine (T2) and rT3 both of which are present in higher quantities in amniotic fluid and cord blood.[28-30]

■ **What is hypoparathyroidism?**

It is a disease caused by deficiency of parathormone that is most commonly seen following subtotal or total thyroidectomy.

■ **What are the chemical findings in hypoparathyroidism?**

The findings are a low serum calcium level associated with a high serum phosphorus level and a low excretion of calcium and phosphorus in the urine associated with a normal ALP level.

■ **What is hyperparathyroidism?**

Hyperparathyroidism is a disease state in which there is overproduction of parathormone caused primarily by hyperplasia or adenoma of the parathyroid gland. It may be caused secondarily by chronic renal insufficiency.

■ **How is the laboratory diagnosis of hyperparathyroidism made?**

The presence of increased serum calcium with an associated low serum phosphate level, increased amounts of calcium and phosphate in the urine, and increases in serum ALP indicates hyperparathyroidism. When associated with increased calcium, an elevated parathormone level is the single best indication of hyperparathyroidism. Increases in proline, hydroxyproline, and cyclic AMP in the urine are other manifestations of hyperparathyroidism.

■ **Is an elevated parathormone value all that is required for a diagnosis of hyperparathyroid disease?**

No. The parathormone determinations must be coupled with calcium studies. In primary hyperparathyroidism, parathormone and calcium are both increased. In renal disease (secondary hyperparathyroidism), the parathormone values are high but the calcium level is low, and in malignancy, the calcium level is high and the parathormone values are low.[31-32]

■ **Is hyperparathyroidism the only disease that can cause an elevated calcium level?**

No. Elevated serum calcium levels may be seen in the milk-alkali syndrome, vitamin D intoxication, sarcoidosis, multiple myeloma, metastatic carcinoma usually involving bone, thyrotoxicosis, and disuse atrophy or osteoporosis. In these instances, however, the serum calcium level is elevated but the parathormone levels are low.

■ **What laboratory determinations are helpful in diagnosing polycystic disease of the ovary (Stein-Leventhal syndrome)?**

High plasma LH levels associated with unusually low FSH levels are noted in polycystic disease. This results from the fact that in the polycystic ovary syndrome, estrogen secretion is maintained and inhibits pituitary FSH.

■ **Can endocrine syndromes be caused by cancer of nonendocrine organs?**

Yes. Gonadotropinlike hormone has been measured in patients with lung cancer of all types. HCGlike hormone has been recorded in association with carcinoma of the lung, liver, breast, and renal cell and with malignant melanoma. ACTHlike hormone has been reported most commonly with oat-cell tumors of the bronchus but has also been seen with tumors of the thymus and pancreas. TSHlike hormone has been associated with trophoblastic tumors and tumors of the testes. Parathyroidlike hormone has been detected with cancer of the lung, kidney, uterus, ovary, and gastrointestinal tract.

Electrolytes

GORDON E. LANG and JOAN SHROUT

■ **Discuss the distribution of water in the human body.**

Water composes approximately 50% to 70% of the weight of the body. The percentage varies inversely with the amount of adipose tissue present and is located in several compartments: (1) intracellular fluid—30% to 35% of the body weight or 55% of the total body water is located within the cells, and (2) extracellular fluid—25% to 30% of the body weight or 45% of the total body water is located outside of the cells. The extracellular fluid is located in several subcompartments: (1) plasma water—about 4.5% of body weight, (b) interstitial fluid and lymph—about 12% of body weight, (c) dense connective tissue, cartilage, and bone water—about 9% of body weight, and (d) transcellular water—about 1.5% of body weight. This is water formed by the secretory cells of the gastrointestinal and respiratory tracts, skin, kidney, brain, thyroid, and gonads.

Water is dynamic as it moves from one compartment to another. Dehydration and water overload are reflected in all compartments.

■ **Discuss the sources of body water and the routes of normal and abnormal water loss.**

The major source of water is that ingested by the oral route. This normally amounts to 1,500 to 3,000 ml/day. A second source is water obtained from oxidation of foodstuff. Oxidation of 100 calories of a mixed diet generates 12 ml of water. Oxidation of body tissues produces about 300 to 400 ml/day.

Water loss is divided into sensible and insensible loss. The normal daily sensible loss consists of about 15 ml of urine per kilogram of body weight and about 100 ml of fecal water. The normal daily insensible loss from the lungs and skin amounts to about 15 ml of water per kilogram of body weight.

Abnormal losses of water occur in periods of increased activity and during certain disease states. Normally about 8,000 ml of digestive juices are secreted into the gastrointestinal tract, and all but 100 ml are reabsorbed. Abnormal losses of gastrointestinal fluid occur in conditions that result in diarrhea and vomiting or after gastrointestinal drainage procedures. An abnormal amount of insensible water loss occurs during fever or when the environmental temperature is increased above 85° F. Abnormal losses of water also occur in renal diseases in which the concentrating ability is reduced.

Measurement of water loss or gain is simple, because any acute gain or loss of body weight represents gain or loss of water. An acute weight change of 1 kilogram represents a gain or loss of 1 liter of water.

■ **What are the plasma electrolytes?**

The principle plasma electrolytes are the cations (sodium, potassium, magnesium, and calcium) and the anions (chloride, bicarbonate, phosphate, sulfate, organic acids, and protein). The concentration of these substances is expressed in mEq/liter. The concentration of proteins in mEq/liter is obtained by multiplying their concentration in gm/dl by the conversion factor 2.43. The mean concentration of the plasma electrolytes is given in Table 11.

■ **What is SI? How does this system of nomenclature affect electrolytes and blood gases?**

SI is the acronym for Le Système Internationale d'Unités. The units of measure are all derived from seven basic units for physical properties: meter (length), kilogram (mass), mole (amount of substance), second (time), ampere (electric current), kelvin or degree Celsius (temperature), and candela (luminous intensity).

SI nomenclature affects or will affect every area of the laboratory, and it is already being used in current literature relating to electrolytes and blood gases. However, SI units have not been adopted by chemists in the United States.

Electrolytes are reported in mmol/liter rather than mEq/liter, except for protein. Gas pressures are reported in pascals, abbreviated Pa or kPa. Various parameters are described in abbreviated form. For example, cd CO_2 (aB) is translated: "concentration (italicized, slanted) of dissolved (regular lowercase 'd') CO_2 in arterial blood." In handwritten or typed descriptions where italicized type is not available, the letter is underlined, e.g., "$\underline{c}$d CO_2 (aB)" or "$\underline{p}CO_2$."

■ **What is meant by "anion-cation balance"?**

Table 11 indicates that the sum of the concentrations of plasma cations (in mEq/liter) is equal to the sum of the concentrations of plasma anions (in mEq/liter). This electroneutrality exists at all times, and its evaluation is useful to maintain quality control on electrolyte determinations and to aid the overall evaluation of patients.

Weisberg has popularized this evaluation using the following formula: $[Na^+] + [K^+] + 7 = [Cl^-] + [HCO_3^-] + 25$. The 7 represents the normal concentration of calcium and magnesium in mEq/liter, whereas the 25 represents the concentration of the unmeasured anions, $HPO_4^=$, $SO_4^=$, organic acids, and protein. Normal anion-cation balance is indicated if the sums of the cations and the anions are within 10 mEq/liter of each other, and with increasing instrument precision, limits of ±5 are reasonable. Abnormal anion-cation balance is indicated when the difference in the sums is greater than 10 mEq/liter. This requires evaluation and explanation before the results are reported. If a laboratory error can be excluded, an abnormality in the unmeasured anions and/or cations exists.

■ **What is indicated by anion-cation imbalance?**

Severe illness is suggested when the sum of the cations is 10 or

Table 11. Concentration of plasma electrolytes

Cations(+)	mEq/liter	Anions(−)	mEq/liter
Sodium (Na⁺)	142	Bicarbonate (HCO₃⁻)	27
Potassium (K⁺)	5	Chloride (Cl⁻)	103
Calcium (Ca⁺⁺)	5	Phosphate (HPO₄⁼)	2
Magnesium (Mg⁺⁺)	2	Sulfate (SO₄⁼)	1
TOTAL	154	Organic acids	5
		Protein	16
		TOTAL	154

more mEq/liter greater than the sum of the anions. This finding usually indicates a marked increase in the unmeasured anions. Four disease states (diabetic ketoacidosis, renal acidosis, lactic acidosis, and salicylate intoxication) should be immediately considered. Diabetic ketoacidosis is indicated by the presence of increased ketones in the serum. Renal acidosis is suggested by elevation of the urea nitrogen, creatinine, and phosphate levels. Lactic acidosis is readily recognized by an increase in the lactic acid. Salicylate intoxication can also be rapidly diagnosed by screening for salicylates in the serum, utilizing a ferric nitrate solution. The latter condition occasionally occurs unrecognized in the pediatric age group.

Illnesses in which the sum of the anions is 10 or more mEq/liter greater than that of the cations are generally of a chronic debilitating nature and most commonly are explained by severe hypoproteinemia. This can also be rapidly identified by determining the total protein with a refractometer. Severe hypercalcemia and hypermagnesemia are other conditions in which the anions may be 10 or more mEq/liter greater than the cations.

Only by rapid evaluation as described above can we assure quality control and give the best possible assistance to the physician in proper evaluation of patients.

■ **What is osmolality?**

Osmolality is a measurement of the total solute concentration of a fluid and represents the number of particles dissolved in 1 kilogram of plasma or urine water.

A solution containing particles equal to Avogadro's number (6.02×10^{23}) in 1 kilogram of solvent contains 1 osmol of solute and has an osmolality of 1. The unit used to describe osmolality of body fluid is the milliosmol (mOsm), which is $1/1,000$ of an osmol.

■ **Discuss calculated osmolality of blood.**

Holmes' formula can be used to calculate osmolality of blood:

$$mOsm/kg = 1.86 \times Na~(mEq/liter) + \frac{Glucose~(mg/dl)}{18} + \frac{Urea~nitrogen~(mg/dl)}{2.8}$$

The amount 1.86 represents the osmotic coefficient for sodium chloride, 18 represents the molecular weight of glucose, and 2.8 represents the molecular weight of urea nitrogen.

To calculate the osmolality, the values for sodium, glucose, and urea nitrogen must be known, as indicated by the above formula. In addition to these three substances, chloride, bicarbonate, and phosphate also contribute significantly to the osmolality and are accounted for by the osmotic coefficient 1.86.

Protein contributes little to total osmolality. To calculate the concentration of protein in mOsm/kg of plasma water, the concentration of protein (gm/dl) is divided by 8. For example, a protein of 8.6 gm/dl is equal to 1.075 mOsm/kg.

With Holmes' formula, the calculated osmolality is usually 5 to 8 mOsm/kg lower than the measured osmolality. A measured osmolality that greatly exceeds the calculated value indicates serious illness characterized by increase in unmeasured solute (e.g., lactic acid, medications, alcohol).

■ **Discuss the clinical value of osmolality.**

The distribution of water between the various fluid compartments is regulated by their osmolality. Hypertonicity of serum will result in cellular dehydration and dilution of the serum by cellular water. Hypotonicity of serum will result in cellular hydration and edema.

The measurement of osmolality is useful in the evaluation of fluid and electrolyte abnormalities, such as the differentiation of the causes of hyponatremia and hypernatremia. The concentrating ability of the kidney is best measured using the urine osmolality rather than specific gravity determinations.

The ratio of urine/serum osmolality is useful in the evaluation of the polyurias and the inappropriate secretion of ADH.

■ **Define and discuss hypokalemia.**

Potassium is the most important intracellular cation. About 98% of the body potassium is located in the intracellular space. It is also present within the extracellular fluid. The normal plasma concentration is 3.5 to 5.5 mEq/liter of plasma. Potassium and sodium help maintain a normal distribution of body water and normal intracellular enzymatic and metabolic reactions.

A plasma potassium concentration of less than 3.5 mEq/liter is known as hypokalemia. A deficit of potassium may be present and not be reflected as a low plasma potassium concentration in some states of hemoconcentration and acidosis. Plasma potassium levels must be interpreted with knowledge of the blood pH. During acidosis, potassium shifts from the intracellular space to the extracellular space, and the hydrogen ion shifts from the extracellular space to to the intracellular space. Generally, plasma potassium concentration rises 0.6 mEq/liter for each 0.1 unit fall in blood pH. Acidosis is therefore associated with an intracellular potassium deficiency and an increase in extracellular potassium.

The kidneys have the ability to conserve sodium and to produce sodium-free urine. They do not, however, have the ability to conserve potassium. When potassium intake is eliminated or significantly reduced, potassium depletion results, because from 20 to 60 mEq/24 hr are eliminated in the urine.

Hypokalemia secondary to an increased renal excretion of potassium occurs in conditions of bicarbonate excess (metabolic alkalosis). Hyperaldosteronism and excessive administration of adrenocortical steroids result in increased potassium excretion and concomitant potassium depletion.

Clinical conditions associated with hypokalemia
1. Abnormal urinary loss of potassium
   a. Overadministration of adrenocortical steroids
   b. Prolonged diuretic therapy (one of the most common causes)
   c. Primary aldosteronism
   d. Cushing's disease
   e. Renal tubular acidosis (inability of renal tubules to maintain a hydrogen ion gradient across the tubular membrane, with substitution of potassium for the hydrogen ion in the sodium reabsorption exchange mechanisms
   f. Diabetic ketoacidosis (occurs following correction of acidosis without administration of potassium)
   g. Respiratory acidosis
   h. Hepatic insufficiency
   i. Starvation and malnutrition
2. Abnormal gastrointestinal loss
   a. Vomiting
   b. Malabsorption syndromes
   c. Diarrhea
   d. Enemas
3. Shift of potassium from serum to cells
   a. Periodic familial paralysis (a rare condition with intermittent attacks of skeletal muscle paralysis)
   b. Extracorporeal perfusion (cardiopulmonary bypass)

■ **Define and indicate some clinical causes of hyperkalemia.**

A plasma potassium concentration of more than 5.5 mEq/liter is known as hyperkalemia. Inadequate renal excretion of potassium is the most frequent cause of hyperkalemia. This occurs during oliguria or anuria in acute and chronic renal failure of almost any cause. Decreased potassium excretion and hyperkalemia also occur in adrenal insufficiency (Addison's disease). As discussed earlier, hyperkalemia may be present in conditions of severe acidosis. Hyperkalemia has been reported in a condition known as malignant hyperthermia, which is hyperpyrexia associated with the administration of various anesthetic agents and the muscle relaxant succinylcholine.

Pseudohyperkalemia is present in certain individuals with thrombocytosis. This is an artificial increase in serum potassium caused by the release of potassium from platelets during the clotting process. This can be avoided by using only heparinized plasma for electrolyte determinations. Hemolysis will falsely increase plasma potassium, as will prolonged contact of plasma with the red cells.

■ **Define and discuss hyponatremia.**

Sodium is the most important cation of the extracellular fluid; its concentration exceeds that of all of the other cations. The normal plasma sodium concentration is 135 to 145 mEq/liter. Sodium is present in a much lower concentration within the intracellular fluid. Sodium is important in the maintenance of normal water distribution. Along with chloride and bicarbonate, it regulates acid-base metabolism. Sodium also functions to maintain normal neuromuscular irritability.

Hyponatremia is a condition in which the plasma sodium concentration is less than 130 mEq/liter. A decrease in the plasma sodium results in a lowering of the osmolality. This inhibits the secretion of ADH from the posterior pituitary gland, causing excretion of water and thus an increase in the plasma sodium concentration. Hypernatremia, conversely, results in an increase in plasma osmolality, causing release of ADH, which promotes retention of water. Generally, hyponatremia results from an excessive amount of water intake, a loss of sodium without a proportional loss of water, or internal shifts of water and electrolytes.

Clinical conditions associated with hyponatremia
I. Pseudohyponatremia
  A. Laboratory error (quality control measures should eliminate most of this type)
  B. Displacement of water. Electrolyte tests are normally performed on plasma or serum, the water content of which varies from 91% to 93%. This percentage may be significantly reduced whenever hyperlipemia or hyperproteinemia is present. Since sodium concentration is expressed as mEq/liter of plasma and not mEq/liter of plasma water, the sodium concentration will be reduced. A normal sodium concentration in a grossly lipemic plasma gives an elevated sodium value. The plasma osmolality is normal in this type of hyponatremia.
II. Dilutional hyponatremia
  A. Water excess
    1. Exogenous (acute—self-inflicted or iatrogenic; intravenous fluids, enemas, etc.)
    2. Endogenous
      a. Features of inappropriate secretion of ADH

(1) Hyponatremia and low serum osmolality
(2) Hypertonic urine that may contain considerable amounts of sodium
(3) Absence of azotemia (normal renal function)
(4) Normal blood volume, so that antidiuresis is not being caused by extracellular volume depletion
(5) Hyponatremia and hypernaturia corrected following fluid restriction
(6) Occurrence:
    (a) Postoperatively in the elderly
    (b) In patients with certain malignant tumors that occasionally secrete ADH-like substances (lung, duodenum, pancreas)
    (c) In certain central nervous system disorders
    (d) In diseases of the lung (pneumonia, TB)
  b. Idiopathic (present in long-standing heart or liver failure, probably related to excessive renal proximal reabsorption of water)

B. Accumulation of nonelectrolyte solutes in the extracellular fluid (hyperosmolality). The accumulation of glucose and/or urea nitrogen in the extracellular fluid results in an osmotic gradient between the cells and the interstitial fluid. This gradient causes a shift of water from the intracellular to the extracellular compartment, resulting in hyponatremia and overall dilution of the hyperosmolar extracellular fluid. Each 35 mg/dl increase in extracellular glucose and each 5 mg/dl increase in urea nitrogen results in 1 mEq/liter decrease in extracellular fluid (plasma) sodium. This type of hyponatremia is seen in uncontrolled diabetes mellitus and in azotemic states.

C. True sodium depletion—hyponatremia caused by sodium loss occurs following:
1. Renal loss—osmotic diuresis, after diuretic therapy, in renal disease, in adrenal insufficiency
2. Gastrointestinal loss—vomiting, diarrhea, nasogastric suction
3. Cutaneous loss—perspiration (excessive), burns
4. Loss of body fluids secondary to thoracentesis or paracentesis
5. Hemorrhage

■ Define and discuss hypernatremia.

Hypernatremia is a condition in which the plasma sodium level is greater than 150 mEq/liter of plasma. It usually results from inadequate intake of water or excessive water loss. Hypernatremia leads to hyperosmolar states, which result in cellular dehydration.

Hypernatremia occurs after deficient water intake, an excessive output of water (such as occurs in diabetes insipidus and protracted vomiting or diarrhea), and cerebral trauma with loss of ADH control. It may also occur iatrogenically after excessive administration of hypertonic sodium chloride solutions.

■ Discuss chloride shift.

Hemoglobin is one of the important buffers responsible for the maintenance of a normal blood pH. Oxyhemoglobin (HbO) is a stronger acid than "reduced" hemoglobin (HHb). The formation of HbO from HHb in the erythrocytes located in the lungs results in the release of H^+, which reacts with HCO_3^- to form carbonic acid

(H_2CO_3). Under the influence of carbonic anhydrase, the H_2CO_3 is converted to H_2O and CO_2. The latter is released to the alveolar air and expired. At the same time, HCO_3^- from the plasma enters the erythrocyte. Chloride, in response, shifts from the erythrocyte to the plasma (the so-called chloride shift).

HHb is formed from HbO on release of O_2 to the tissues. CO_2 produced in the tissues enters the erythrocytes, where under the influence of the enzyme carbonic anhydrase, H_2CO_3 is formed. The latter is ionized to form H^+ and HCO_3^-. The reduced Hb reacts with the H^+ to form HHb. Some of the HCO_3^- that is formed enters the plasma, resulting in a shift of the chloride from the plasma to the erythrocyte. Therefore, arterial plasma has a higher chloride level than does venous plasma.

■ **What is an acid? What is a base?**

According to the Brønsted theory, an acid is a proton (hydrogen ion, H^+) donor. A base is a proton acceptor.

$$H_2CO_3 \rightleftharpoons HCO_3^- + H^+$$
Acid   Base

■ **What is an anion? What is a cation?**

An anion is a negatively charged ion, e.g., Cl^-, that migrates in an electrical field to the anode. A cation is a positively charged ion, e.g., Na^+, that migrates in an electrical field to the cathode.

■ **Define pH.**

pH is a simplified expression of hydrogen ion concentration and is equal to the negative logarithm of the hydrogen ion concentration. A decreasing pH represents an increasing H^+ concentration. A 0.3 unit decrease in the pH is equivalent to a doubling of the H^+ concentration.

pH	$[H^+]$
7.10	80 nmol/liter
7.40	40 nmol/liter
7.70	20 nmol/liter

The normal ranges are 7.32 to 7.42 (venous) and 7.35 to 7.45 (arterial).

■ **Define P_{CO_2}.**

P_{CO_2} is the partial pressure of CO_2 in a gas phase in equilibrium with liquid blood. It is a measurement of respiratory function that indicates the adequacy of ventilation. The term "hypercapnia" indicates hypoventilation, which results in an elevated P_{CO_2}. Hypocapnia indicates hyperventilation, which results in a low P_{CO_2}. The normal P_{CO_2} ranges are 42 to 55 torr (venous) and 34 to 46 torr (arterial).

■ **What is the Henderson-Hasselbalch equation?**

The Henderson-Hasselbalch equation is an expression of the fundamental relation of physiologic acid-base chemistry; it is written as follows:

$$pH = pK + \log \frac{base}{acid} \qquad (1)$$

For the carbonic acid–bicarbonate system it is written:

$$pH = 6.1 + \log \frac{[HCO_3^-]\ mEq/liter}{[H_2CO_3]\ mEq/liter} \qquad (2)$$

where

6.1 = pK of H_2CO_3 at 38° C in serum

pH should be thought of as simply the ratio $[HCO_3^-]: [H_2CO_3]$. The pH is directly proportional to this ratio. For example, the ratio resulting in a pH of 7.40 is 20:1.

If any two of the values pH, $[HCO_3^-]$, or $[H_2CO_3]$ are known, the third value can be readily calculated. The $[H_2CO_3]$ is obtainable from the P_{CO_2}, because the $[H_2CO_3]$ is directly proportional to the P_{CO_2}.

$$[H_2CO_3] = 0.03 \times P_{CO_2} \qquad (3)$$

where

0.03 = Solubility coefficient of CO_2 at 37° C relating $[H_2CO_3]$ to P_{CO_2}

The availability of direct measurements of pH and P_{CO_2} and the above equation allow for the calculation of other values—HCO_3^-, H_2CO_3, and total CO_2. Nomograms of Siggaard-Anderson and Weisberg or the utilization of minicomputers, such as those produced by Olivetti, Wang, and others, simplifies the calculation.

■ **Define buffer base.**

Buffer base is the sum of the concentrations in mEq/liter of the buffer anions of whole blood: bicarbonate, phosphate, hemoglobin, and plasma protein. The normal range is 46 to 50 mEq/liter.

■ **Define base excess.**

Base excess (BE) is equal to the actual buffer base minus the normal buffer base (defined above). The actual determination of BE is not practical, but it can readily be determined using the Siggaard-Anderson alignment nomogram when pH, P_{CO_2}, and hemoglobin are known. If a programmable calculator is available, BE can also be calculated using the following equation of Alvin P. Long, Jr.:

$$BE = \left[1 - \frac{Hb}{75}\right][HCO_3^- - 23.94] + [11.4 + 1.323\ Hb][pH - 7.4]$$

The normal range is -2.5 to $+2.5$ mEq/liter.

For practical purposes, BE is a measurement of bicarbonate excess or deficit. A positive result indicates metabolic alkalosis (bicarbonate excess) and a negative value below the normal range indicates metabolic acidosis (bicarbonate deficit).

■ **List and define several terms that have been used to describe CO_2.**

Total CO_2, or CO_2 content, represents the sum of the bicarbonate, carbonic acid, and dissolved carbon dioxide that is present in blood drawn anaerobically. Total CO_2 can be best determined by calculation using the Henderson-Hasselbalch equation when pH and PCO_2 are known. Direct measurements using the Van Slyke blood gas apparatus or the Natelson microgasometer have been performed in the past before the advent of modern blood gas analyzers.

CO_2 combining power and *CO_2 capacity* measure the carbon dioxide of separated or true plasma following equilibration to a PCO_2 of 40 torr. After correction for dissolved CO_2 (i.e., H_2CO_3), it represents bicarbonate. These values are only of historical interest.

Bicarbonate is the $[HCO_3^-]$ in anaerobically drawn blood and is best determined by calculation using the Henderson-Hasselbalch equation.

Standard bicarbonate was defined by Jorgensen and Astrup as the plasma bicarbonate concentration in fully oxygenated blood at 38° C when the PCO_2 is 40 torr. This value was popular before the development of the direct PCO_2 electrode and was derived utilizing the Astrup method and apparatus.

■ **What are the minimum data required to adequately evaluate a clinical acid-base disorder?**

A measurement of pH, PCO_2, and HCO_3^- is the minimum data necessary to adequately evaluate and manage a clinical acid-base disorder. CO_2, measured by whatever method, without pH and PCO_2 is insufficient not only to evaluate an acid-base disorder but also to uncover a disorder when it exists. A "normal" total CO_2 content of 27 mEq/liter can occur with a pH of 6.80, 7.80, or anywhere in between. This is analogous to informing a visitor to Washington, D.C. that the White House is on Pennsylvania Avenue, with the result that he arrives at the Capitol or at the I.R.S. Office. It is essential to provide routine pH, Pco_2, and HCO_3^- measurements on all requests for CO_2. It is valid to perform these determinations under all circumstances on properly drawn venous blood.

■ **How are blood pH and Pco_2 measured?**

pH, or $[H^+]$, is determined potentiometrically using a hydrogen ion–sensitive glass electrode that contains an Ag/AgCl wire immersed in an electrolyte of fixed pH. An electrical potential is created when a glass membrane separates two solutions of different $[H^+]$. This potential is compared with a reference voltage supplyed by an Hg/Hg_2Cl_2 (calomel) electrode that is connected to the unknown sample and the glass electrode by a solution of saturated KCl. The membrane potential is proportional to the log $[H^+]$.

Pco_2 is also measured potentiometrically. The Pco_2 electrode is a combination pH/reference electrode that is covered with a membrane that is permeable to nonionized molecules such as CO_2 gas but not to ions such as $[H^+]$. A thin layer of a bicarbonate solution is located between the membrane and the electrode. The pH of the bicarbonate solution changes in response to CO_2, which diffuses into it from the sample being measured. The change in pH of the bicarbonate solution is exponentially related to the Pco_2 of the sample being measured.

■ **Discuss the four classic types of acid-base imbalance.**

Acid-base disturbances are best described by indicating the alteration in the $[HCO_3^-] : [H_2CO_3]$ ratio. Traditionally, abnormalities in the $[HCO_3^-]$ have been called metabolic, and abnormalities in the $[H_2CO_3]$ have been called respiratory. The metabolic component, $[HCO_3^-]$, is regulated primarily by renal mechanisms, whereas the respiratory component, Pco_2, is regulated by the lungs. Renal and pulmonary mechanisms attempt to maintain a 20:1 bicarbonate–carbonic acid ratio by retaining or eliminating HCO_3^- or H_2CO_3 (Pco_2) respectively.

Bicarbonate excess, or metabolic alkalosis, is a disorder in which the concentration of bicarbonate is increased, resulting in an increase in the bicarbonate–carbonic acid ratio. The decrease in $[H^+]$ results in hypoventilation and an increase in Pco_2 ($[H_2CO_3]$). Renal mechanisms are also stimulated to increase bicarbonate excretion, resulting in a decrease in $[HCO_3^-]$. Common causes for this disorder are vomiting, loss of gastric acid by suction, administration of various diuretic agents, hypokalemia of any cause, and overadministration of alkali such as sodium bicarbonate.

Bicarbonate deficit, or metabolic acidosis, is a disorder in which the concentration of bicarbonate is decreased, resulting in a decrease in the bicarbonate–carbonic acid ratio. The increase in $[H^+]$ results in hyperventilation and a decrease in Pco_2 ($[H_2CO_3]$). Renal mechanisms are also activated so as to retain HCO_3^-. Common causes for this disorder are diabetes mellitus, lactic acidosis, salicylate intoxication (late), renal failure, and overadministration of acidifying agents such as NH_4Cl.

Carbonic acid excess, or respiratory acidosis, is a hypoventilatory disorder in which the concentration of carbonic acid is increased ($\uparrow Pco_2$), resulting in a decrease in the bicarbonate–carbonic acid ratio. Compensatory renal mechanisms are slowly activated in response to the increased Pco_2, resulting in retention of HCO_3^-. Secondarily, ventilation is increased in response to an elevated Pco_2 and a decreased pH. Common causes of hypoventilation are central nervous system depression of any cause, such as CNS trauma and use of certain drugs; acute mechanical obstruction of the airway; and chronic obstructive pulmonary disease.

Carbonic acid deficit, or respiratory alkalosis, is a hyperventilatory disorder in which the concentration of carbonic acid is decreased ($\downarrow Pco_2$), resulting in an increase in the bicarbonate–carbonic acid ratio. Compensation is generally slow unless the cause is alleviated. Although there is some increase in renal excretion of bicarbonate following prolonged hyperventilation, a considerable proportion of the decreased HCO_3^- is secondary to a lactic acidosis that occurs as a result of tissue hypoxia. The hypoxia is secondary to a shift to the left in the oxygen dissociation curve that occurs following a rise in pH. Common causes are psychogenic hyperventilation; respiratory center stimulation such as occurs early in salicylate intoxication, fever, and anoxia; hepatic failure; and iatrogenic causes secondary to mechanical hyperventilation.

It should be remembered that compensation for an acid-base disorder only occurs if the organ (lung or kidney) responsible is functionally able to respond to the primary disorder. When compensation cannot occur, the patient is in jeopardy.

Occasionally two primary acid-base imbalances, one respiratory and one metabolic, occur simultaneously in the same patient. For example, a patient with chronic obstructive pulmonary disease who develops acute diabetic ketoacidosis has a mixed imbalance (primary carbonic acid excess and primary bicarbonate deficit). These individuals are seriously ill and can readily die, because it is difficult if not impossible for them to compensate. Combinations of imbalance states are possible; Weisberg, for example, has identified 13 states.

■ **Discuss the composition of atmospheric air.**

The total pressure exerted by a gas mixture such as atmospheric air is simply the sum of the partial pressure of all the gases present in the mixture. The barometric pressure (BP) at sea level is about 760 torr. BP decreases with altitude: at 18,000 feet it is one half of that at sea level. Dry atmospheric air contains 20.93% oxygen, 0.03% carbon dioxide, 79.4% nitrogen, and traces of gases, such as argon. The percent composition is the same at all altitudes. To calculate the partial pressure of various gases, the percent is multiplied by the BP.

Air that enters the respiratory tree is rapidly saturated with water vapor, which exerts a partial pressure of 47 torr at 37° C. (The symbol for partial pressure is capital P followed by the gas being discussed. In SI nomenclature, an italicized p is used, and the unit is kPa; 0.133 kPa = 1 torr.) Therefore, dry atmospheric air at sea level will have a BP of 760–47 or 713 torr.

The partial pressures of dry atmospheric air as it enters the respiratory tree are:

$$P_{O_2} = 0.2093 \times 713 = 149 \text{ torr}$$
$$P_{CO_2} = 0.003 \times 713 = 0.2 \text{ torr}$$
$$P_{N_2} = 0.7904 \times 713 = 564 \text{ torr}$$

■ **Discuss the composition of the air in the alveoli of the lungs.**

The body is continually using oxygen and producing carbon dioxide; therefore, the partial pressure of oxygen in the alveolar air (PA_{O_2}) and in the tissues will be lower than atmospheric air, and the partial pressure of carbon dioxide (PA_{CO_2}) will be higher. The exact composition is a function of the composition of the inspired air, the rate of carbon dioxide production, and the ventilatory rate and volume. When one breathes room air, the sum of the PA_{O_2} and PA_{CO_2} is fixed, and any change results in an equal and opposite change in the other. A 10, 20, or 40 torr rise in PA_{CO_2} will result in a 10, 20, or 40 torr decrease in PA_{CO_2}. The average PA_{CO_2} is 40 torr, and the average PA_{O_2} is 100 torr.

■ **Discuss the exchange of gases in the lungs and in the tissues.**

The exchange of gases in the lungs through the alveolar membrane occurs by diffusion into the blood or in a reverse direction, depending on the difference in the partial pressure of each gas on either side of the alveolar membrane. The diffusibility of CO_2 is twenty times that of O_2. This fact helps explain the presence of a normal Pa_{CO_2} or a very low Pa_{O_2} in some individuals with thickened alveolar membranes , as occurs in interstitial pneumonitis.

The normal exchange of oxygen and carbon dioxide in the lungs occurs as follows:

PA_{O_2} (alveolar air) = 100 torr
Pv_{O_2} (proximal alveolar capillary) = 40 torr

The 60-torr pressure gradient drives oxygen into the alveolar capillary blood from the alveoli.

PA_{CO_2} (alveolar air) = 40 torr
Pv_{CO_2} (proximal alveolar capillary) = 46 torr

The 6-torr pressure gradient and rapid diffusability of carbon dioxide drive it from the alveolar capillary blood into the alveoli.

Oxygen and carbon dioxide present in tissue capillary blood diffuse through the capillary membrane into the tissues or in a reverse direction, depending on the difference in pressure of the gas in question on either side of the membrane. The normal exchange of oxygen and carbon dioxide in the tissues occurs as follows:

Pa_{O_2} (proximal tissue capillary, arterial) = 100 torr
Po_2 tissue = 30 torr
Pv_{O_2} (distal tissue capillary, venous) = 40 torr

The 70-torr pressure gradient drives oxygen from the capillary blood into the tissue, from where it is returned to the lungs for reoxygenation.

Pa_{CO_2} (proximal tissue capillary, arterial) = 40 torr
Pco_2 tissue = 50 torr
Pv_{CO_2} (distal tissue capillary, venous) = 46 torr

The 10-torr pressure gradient and rapid diffusibility of carbon dioxide drive it from the tissue into the distal venous capillaries.

■ **Discuss the transportation of oxygen by blood.**

Oxygen is transported from the lungs to the tissue in the form of oxygen-bound hemoglobin and oxygen dissolved in the plasma water. Only a small amount, 0.3 ml of oxygen per deciliter of blood, is carried in the dissolved state when atmospheric air is breathed. Each gram of hemoglobin when fully saturated with oxygen will combine with 1.34 ml of oxygen. Hemoglobin is almost fully saturated with oxygen when Po_2 is about 100 torr. The *oxygen capacity* of blood is defined as the amount of oxygen chemically combined with a deciliter of blood when the hemoglobin is fully saturated. It is readily calculated by multiplying the hemoglobin in gm/dl by 1.34. A person with a hemoglobin of

15 gm/dl will have an oxygen capacity of 20.1 ml/dl ($15 \times 1.34 = 20.1$). *Oxygen content* is the quantity of oxygen actually combined with hemoglobin.

The ratio of oxygen content to oxygen capacity multiplied by 100 is known as *percent oxygen saturation*. The percent saturation of hemoglobin is related to Po_2. This relationship is readily understood if expressed graphically by plotting percent saturation on the ordinate and Po_2 on the abscissa. The curve obtained is called the *oxygen dissociation curve*. The curve is sigmoid in shape because the amount of oxygen bound to hemoglobin is not linearly related to Po_2. As the Po_2 decreases, the percent saturation decreases slowly until the tension is about 50 to 55 torr, at which point oxygen is rapidly released from hemoglobin. This is important in that there must be a considerable reduction in the Po_2 of inspired air before any significant change in saturation occurs. As blood flows through the tissues that have a lower Po_2, oxygen is released until the Po_2 of the arterial blood approaches that of the tissue. Normally the Pa_{O_2} is reduced from 100 torr to 40 torr, resulting in release of one third of the oxygen to the tissues. This provides a two-thirds reserve of oxygenated blood in the event that there is a reduction in oxygen in the inspired air.

■ **Discuss some factors that affect the dissociation of oxyhemoglobin.**

The configuration of the oxygen dissociation curve is described by the P_{50}. P_{50} is the Po_2 at which hemoglobin is 50% saturated. The normal P_{50} at a pH of 7.40 and a temperature of 37° C is about 27 torr. Several factors, namely, temperature, pH, Pco_2, and the quantity of red cell 2,3-diphosphoglycerate (2,3-DPG), affect the dissociation of hemoglobin. An increase in P_{50} or a shift to the right of the oxygen dissociation curve indicates that the affinity of hemoglobin for oxygen is decreased and that the ability of hemoglobin to release oxygen to the tissues at a given Po_2 is increased. A decrease in P_{50} or a shift to the left of the oxygen dissociation curve indicates that the affinity of hemoglobin is increased and that its ability to release oxygen to the tissues at a given Po_2 is decreased.

It has long been known that a decrease in pH, an increase in Pco_2, and hyperthermia cause a shift to the right of the oxygen dissociation curve, whereas an increase in pH, a decrease in Pco_2, and hypothermia result in a shift to the left. Recent studies have shown that the position of the oxygen dissociation curve of adult hemoglobin is also affected by the interaction of hemoglobin with red cell organic phosphates. About 80% of the organic phosphates in the red cell consists of

2,3-DPG, a normal glycolytic intermediate of the Embden-Meyerhof cycle. ATP constitutes most of the remainder of the organic phosphates.

Red cell 2,3-DPG and the P_{50} are increased in clinical conditions in which there is an increase in oxygen demand or oxygen lack, as in chronic lung disease, cyanotic heart disease, anemias secondary to iron deficiency, and red cell pyruvate kinase deficiency. It is also increased after vigorous exercise and during adaptation to high altitudes.

Red cell 2,3-DPG and P_{50} are decreased after massive transfusion of stored blood, after septic shock, in neonatal respiratory distress syndrome, and in carbon monoxide intoxication.

Persistent alkalosis or increased blood pH results in increased production of red cell 2,3-DPG, whereas persistent acidosis or decreased blood pH results in decreased production of red cell 2,3-DPG. These responses counteract the pH effect on the oxygen dissociation curve.

■ **How are Po_2, percent O_2 saturation, and P_{50} measured?**

Po_2 is measured by a Clark electrode, which consists of a platinum cathode and an Ag/AgCl anode. The electrode is connected to an external low-voltage power supply and is covered with a semipermeable membrane. The membrane permits oxygen to pass through to the cathode, where the oxygen is reduced. An electrical current proportional to the Po_2 is generated.

Percent oxygen saturation is now most commonly measured by one of several oximeters that are available. These oximeters determine spectrophotometrically the ratio of oxygenated hemoglobin to total hemoglobin present in a blood sample. The absorbance of the blood sample is measured at two specific wavelengths, one being the isosbestic point, or the wavelength at which oxyhemoglobin and reduced hemoglobin have the same absorbance, and the other being the wavelength at which oxyhemoglobin and reduced hemoglobin have different absorbances. The ratio of the absorbances at these two wavelengths is proportional to the percent oxygen saturation.

Percent saturation and Po_2 can also be calculated from an oxygen dissociation curve if the pH and either the Po_2 or the percent saturation of the blood sample are known. This may be accurate if the P_{50} of the sample is within normal limits; however, when there is a shift to the right or left of the oxygen dissociation curve, the calculated value may be erroneous.

P_{50} is determined by measuring Po_2, percent oxygen saturation, and pH on two aliquots of blood that have been equilibrated at 37° C in a tonometer with two gases of known oxygen content. The percent oxygen saturation of one aliquot should be slightly above 50% saturated and the other slightly below 50% saturated. The P_{50} can then be obtained by plotting the percent saturation against PO_2 corrected to pH 7.40. If a minicomputer is available, P_{50} can be calculated using the Hill equation.

- **Discuss the collection of blood for pH, Pco_2, and Po_2 studies.**

Venous blood, when properly drawn, is satisfactory for electrolyte, pH, and PCO_2 studies under almost all circumstances. Impressions gained from proper interpretation of the results obtained from venous blood will be the same as those obtained from arterial blood. Arterial blood studies are generally required when oxygen measurements are desired in addition to pH and PCO_2.

Medical technologists can and should be taught to obtain both venous and arterial blood so that electrolyte, pH, PCO_2, PO_2, and percent oxygen saturation determinations may be available at all times.

The collection of venous blood for acid-base studies should be done without prolonged venous stasis. The first blood obtained should be used for the determination of pH and PCO_2. If a tourniquet is used to locate a vein, it must not be released until after the blood is obtained, or the pH will be falsely low.

Arterial blood can be readily obtained relatively painlessly without a tourniquet from the brachial, radial, or femoral arteries without the use of local anesthetic agents. After the needle is removed, firm pressure must be applied to the puncture site for 5 minutes.

Heparin is the only satisfactory anticoagulant for these determinations. Blood collection in heparinized glass or plastic syringes or vacuum tubes is satisfactory only for pH and PCO_2 studies. If PO_2 or percent oxygen saturation is desired, blood must be obtained anaerobically in heparinized tight-fitting syringes. The presence of air bubbles that exceed 0.5% to 1% of the volume of blood in the collecting syringe will introduce significant errors in the PO_2. Heparinized vacuum tubes are unsatisfactory for oxygen studies, because they contain sufficient oxygen to substantially affect the PO_2 and percent oxygen saturation.

- **Discuss the effect of the patient's termperature on pH, Pco_2, Po_2, and O_2 saturation.**

The pH of blood is inversely proportional to temperature, and PCO_2

and PO_2 are directly proportional to temperature. The O_2 saturation does not change with temperature.

The temperature of the modern blood gas analyzer is maintained by a thermostat at 37° C (which is the average normal human temperature). When a patient's temperature deviates significantly from 37° C (less than 35° or more than 39° C), the determined values will be significantly different from the actual values. The determined pH is falsely decreased and the PCO_2 and PO_2 are falsely increased if the patient is hypothermic. In hyperthermic states, the determined pH is falsely increased and the PCO_2 and PO_2 are falsely decreased. For example, the pH, PCO_2, and PO_2 of a patient whose temperature is 30° C are determined to be 7.28, 58 torr, and 100 torr, respectively. When correction is made for this 7° C change in temperature, the actual pH, PCO_2, and PO_2 are 7.38, 41 torr, and 67 torr, respectively. The actual pH, PCO_2, and PO_2 can be determined by calculation using various formulas. The newer blood gas analyzers, such as the IL 813, will automatically make these calculations.*

■ **Where is calcium located and what is its function?**

Ninety-nine percent of the body calcium is located in the bones and teeth. Most of the remaining 1% is located in the extracellular fluid. The normal serum calcium is 4.3 to 5.5 mEq/liter. Fifty percent to 60% of serum calcium is ionized or complexed with citrate and other inorganic anions, and the remainder is bound to albumin and beta globulin. The ionized fraction is the physiologically important one.

Calcium is required to maintain bone and tooth development, neuromuscular function, and blood coagulation. It is also required for a variety of enzymatic reactions. Normal cellular membrane function and the maintenance of renal concentrating mechanisms also require this important cation.

■ **How do parathormone and thyrocalcitonin affect the serum calcium level?**

Parathormone (PTH) is a hormone secreted by the parathyroid glands. A reduced serum calcium level stimulates its release from the parathyroid glands. A high serum inorganic phosphorus level, which

---

*Two excellent references containing formulas for these calculations are Ruiz, B. C., Tucker, W. K., and Kirby, R. K.: A program for calculation of intrapulmonary shunts, blood-gas and acid-base values with a programmable calculator, Anesthesiology 42:88-95, 1975; and Kelman, G. R., and Nunn, J. F.: Nomograms for correction of blood PO_2 and PCO_2, pH and base excess for time and temperature, J. Appl. Physiol. 21:1484-1490, 1966.

may be present in chronic renal failure, results in a decrease in serum calcium, which causes excessive secretion of PTH.

PTH stimulates an increased renal excretion of phosphate and a decreased excretion of calcium. It also promotes calcium absorption from the intestine and resorption of calcium and phosphate from the bones, resulting in an increased serum calcium level.

Thyrocalcitonin is a hormone liberated by the parafollicular cells of the thyroid. It counteracts the actions of PTH in that bone resorption of calcium is inhibited and serum calcium level is lowered. Its secretion is stimulated by an elevated serum calcium level.

■ **Define hypercalcemia and list some of its causes. What tests may be used to evaluate hypercalcemia?**

Hypercalcemia is a condition in which the serum calcium concentration is greater than 5.5 mEq/liter.

Clinical conditions associated with hypercalcemia
1. Laboratory error
2. Neoplasia
   a. Metastatic to bone: lymphoma, leukemia, multiple myeloma, breast, lung, kidney, ovary, GI tract
   b. Primary tumors that produce PTH-like substances: hypernephroma, lung
3. Sarcoidosis
4. Hypervitaminosis D
5. Milk-alkali syndrome
6. Hyperparathyroidism
7. Adrenal insufficiency
8. Idiopathic hypercalcemia of infancy
9. Acute skeletal atrophy of disuse
10. Hyperthyroidism

Laboratory tests to evaluate hypercalcemia
1. Repeat serum calcium.
2. Serum inorganic phosphorus
3. Urinary calcium and phosphate excretion
4. Phosphate clearance
5. Tubular reabsorption of phosphate
6. Alkaline phosphatase
7. Cortisone suppression: 100 to 150 mg cortisone per day for 5 to 10 days results in lowering of serum calcium level in most patients except those with primary hyperparathyroidism
8. Radioimmunoassay for PTH

■ **Define hypocalcemia and list some of its causes.**

Hypocalcemia is defined as a condition in which the serum calcium concentration is less than 4.5 mEq/liter. The clinical sign of this condition is neuromuscular irritability (tetany).

Conditions associated with hypocalcemia
1. Laboratory error
2. Vitamin D deficiency—rickets, osteomalacia
3. Steatorrhea—sprue, pancreatic insufficiency
4. Tetany of newborn—secondary to high phosphate intake
5. Hypoparathyroidism—may be temporary following thyroidectomy
6. Pseudohypoparathyroidism—end-organ refractoriness to PTH (Differentiated from true hypoparathyroidism by the Ellsworth-Howard test. The patient is given PTH, and urinary phosphate excretion is measured. Phosphate excretion is increased in hypoparathyroidism but not in pseudohypoparathyroidism.)
7. Renal failure with hyperphosphatemia
8. Pancreatitis, acute
9. Pregnancy with poor intake of calcium

■ **What is the distribution of magnesium and what is its function?**

Magnesium is the fourth most abundant extracellular cation and the second most abundant intracellular cation. Seventy percent of the body magnesium is complexed with calcium and phosphorus in the bones. Thirty-five percent of the plasma magnesium is protein-bound. Magnesium is the only cation that has a higher concentration in the cerebrospinal fluid than in the plasma. The normal serum magnesium is 1.5 to 2.5 mEq/liter.

Magnesium is an activator for many enzyme systems involved in the metabolism of carbohydrates and protein. Magnesium, like calcium, affects neuromuscular irritability.

Magnesium is absorbed by the small intestine. Renal excretion is inhibited by PTH. A low serum magnesium level stimulates the parathyroid to release PTH.

■ **Discuss hypomagnesemia.**

Hypomagnesemia is a condition in which the serum magnesium concentration is less than 1.5 mEq/liter. Magnesium deficiency states occur when there is a deficient intake, when there is poor absorption by the small bowel, or when there is excessive loss from the urinary or gastrointestinal tract. Endocrinologic disorders may also be a cause.

Symptoms may include tetany, seizures, hyperexcitability, and psychotic behavior. Hypomagnesemia may coexist with hypocalcemia or with normocalcemic states. Tetany with hypomagnesemia but normal serum calcium level and pH has been recognized as the "magnesium deficiency–tetany syndrome." The difference between hypocalcemic and hypomagnesemic tetany is determined by measurements of the serum content of these cations.

Hypomagnesemia has been associated with the following disorders: various malabsorption syndromes, alcoholism, both hyper- and hypoparathyroidism, diabetic ketoacidosis, chronic renal disease of various causes, burns, diuretic therapy, pancreatitis, and tumors metastatic to bone.

■ **Define hypermagnesemia.**

Hypermagnesemia is a condition in which the serum magnesium concentration is greater than 2.5 mEq/liter. Hypermagnesemia is most often seen in renal failure or is iatrogenic in nature. It has also been reported in diabetic coma and in patients with megacolon. Coma occurs with magnesium levels above 14 mEq/liter.

References

1. Wilkinson, J. H.: Clinical significance of enzyme activity measurements, Clin. Chem. 16:882-890, Nov. 1970.
2. Posen, S.: Turnover of circulating enzymes, Clin. Chem. 16:71-84, Feb. 1970.
3. Roberts, R., Sobel, B. E., and Parker, C. W.: Radioimmunoassay for creatine kinase isoenzymes, Science 194:855-857, Nov. 19, 1976.
4. Itano, M.: The detection of CPK 1 (BB) in serum; a summary of sixteen cases, Am. J. Clin. Pathol. 65:351-355, March 1976.
5. Asada, M., and Galambos, J. T.: Sorbital dehydrogenase and hepatocellular injury; an experimental and clinical study, Gastroenterology 44:578, 1963.
6. Fishman, W. H.: Perspectives on alkaline phosphatase isoenzymes, Am. J. Med. 56:617-650, May 1974.
7. Yam, L. T.: Clinical significance of the human acid phosphatases; a review, Am. J. Med. 56:604-616, May 1974.
8. Mishkin, S., Bates, J., and others: Possible mechanisms of normal amylase activity in hyperlipemic pancreatitis, Can. Med. J. 115:1016-1019, Nov. 20, 1976.
9. Lesser, P. B., and Warshaw, A. L.: Differentiation of pancreatitis from common bile duct obstruction with hyperamylasemia, Gastroenterology 68:636-641, April 1975.
10. Johnson, S. G., Ellis, C. J., and Levitt, M. D.: Mechanism of increased renal clearance of amylase/creatinine in acute pancreatitis, N. Engl. J. Med. 295:1214-1217, Nov. 25, 1976.
11. Dürr, H. K., Bode, J. C., Lanlisch, P. G., and others: Amylase-creatinine clearance ratio in pancreatitis letter, N. Engl. J. Med. 296:635, March 17, 1977.
12. Lehrner, L. M., Ward, J. C., Karn, R. C., and others: An evaluation of the usefulness of amylase isoenzyme differentiation in patients with hyperamylasemia, Am. J. Clin. Pathol. 66:576-587, Sept. 1976.
13. O'Malley, B. W., and Schrader, W. T.: The receptors of steroid hormones, Sci. Am. 234:32-43, Feb. 1976.
14. Catt, K. J.: ABC of endocrinology. I: Hormones in general, Lancet 1:763-765, April 11, 1970.
15. Marsh, J. M.: The role of cyclic AMP in gonadal steroidogenesis, Bio. Reprod. 14:30-53, Feb. 1976.
16. Knights, E. B., Baylin, S. B., and Foster, G. V.: Control of polypeptide hormones by enzymatic degradation, Lancet 2:719-723, Sept. 19, 1973.
17. Kahn, C. R., Rosen, S. W., Weintraub, B. D., and others: Ectopic production of chorionic gonadotropin and its subunits by islet-cell tumors; a specific marker for malignancy, N. Engl. J. Med. 297:565-569, Sept. 15, 1977.
18. Braunstein, G. D., Vaitukaitis, J. L., Carbone, P. P., and others: Ectopic production

of human chorionic gonadotropin by neoplasms, Ann. Intern. Med. **78:**39-45, Jan. 1973.

19. Ramey, J. N., and Burrow, G. N.: Clinical uses of thyrotropin-releasing hormone, Am. Fam. Physician **12:**93-100, July 1975.

20. DeVane, G. W., Siler, T. M., and Yen, S. S.: Acute suppression of insulin and glucose levels by synthetic somatostatin in normal human subjects, J. Clin. Endocrinol. Metab. **38:**913-915, May 1974.

21. Lin, T., and Tucci, J. R.: Provocative test of growth hormone release, Ann. Intern. Med. **80:**464-469, April 1974.

22. Colburn, W. A.: Radioimmunoassay for cortisol using antibodies against prednisolone conjugated at the 3-position, J. Clin. Endocrinol. Metab. **41:**868-875, Nov. 1975.

23. Chopra, I. J., Williams, D. C., Orgiazzi, J., and others: Opposite effects of dexamethasone on serum concentrations of 3, 3', 5'-triiodothyronine (reverse T3) and 3, 3', 5 triiodothyronine (T3), J. Clin. Endocrinol. Metab. **41:**911-920, Nov. 1975.

24. Chopra, I. J., Sack, J., and Fisher, D. A.: Circulating 3, 3', 5'-triiodothyronine (reverse T3) in the human newborn, J. Clin. Invest. **55:**1137-1141, June 1975.

25. Oliver, C., Charvet, J. P., Codaccioni, J. L., and others: Radioimmunoassay of thyrotropin-releasing hormone (TRH) in human plasma and urine, J. Clin. Endocrinol. Metab. **39:**406-409, Aug. 1974.

26. Erenberg, A., Phelps, D. L., Lam, R., and others: Total and free thyroid hormone concentrations in the neonatal period, Pediatrics **53:**211-216, Feb. 1974.

27. Burman, K. D., Read, J., Dimond, R. C., and others: Measurement of 3, 3', 5'-triiodothyronine (reverse T3), 3, 3'-L-diiodothyronine, T3 and T4 in human amniotic fluid and in cord and maternal serum, J. Clin. Endocrinol. Metab. **43:**1351-1359, Dec. 1976.

28. Chopra, I. J.: A radioimmunoassay for measurement of 3, 3', 5'-triiodothyronine (reverse T3), J. Clin. Invest. **54:**583-592, Sept. 1974.

29. Chopra, I. J., and Crandall, B. F.: Thyroid hormones and thyrotropin in amniotic fluids, N. Engl. J. Med. **293:**740-743, Oct. 9, 1975.

30. Mitchell, M. L., Larson, P. R., Harvey, L. L., and others: Screening for congenital hypothyroidism; results in the newborn population of New England, J.A.M.A. **239:**2348-2351, 1978.

31. Benson, R. C., Jr., Riggs, B. L., Pickard, B. M., and others: Radioimmunoassay of parathyroid hormone in hypercalcemic patients with malignant disease, Am. J. Med. **56:**821-826, June 1974.

32. Brewer, H. B., Jr., Fairwell, T., Roman, R., and others: Human parathyroid hormone; amino-acid sequence of the amino-terminal residues 1-34, Proc. Natl. Acad. Sci. U.S.A. **69:**3585-3588, Dec. 1972.

Recommended readings

Batsakis, J. G., Briere, R. O., and Merker, S. F.: Diagnostic enzymology, Chicago, 1970, American Society of Clinical Pathologists.

Martin, J. B., Reichlin, S., and Brown, G. M.: Clinical neuroendocrinology, Philadelphia, 1977, F. A. Davis Co.

Mattenheimer, H.: Clinical enzymology, Ann Arbor, Mich., 1971, Ann Arbor Science Publishers, Inc.

Tietz, N. M., editor: Fundamentals of clinical chemistry, Philadelphia, 1976, W. B. Saunders Co.

Wolf, P. L., Williams, D., and Vonder Muehll, E.: Practical clinical enzymology, New York, 1973, John Wiley & Sons, Inc.

Index

A

ABO blood group system
  genotype determination, 49
  inheritance, 49-50
  isoagglutinins, 49
  major groups, 44
  "naturally occurring" antibodies, 45
  phenotypes, 50
Absolute monocytosis, 26
Absorption spectrophotometry, 133
Accuracy, 144
Acetic acid, 114
Acid, 196
Acid phosphatase, 165
Acid-base disorder, 198-199
Acid-base imbalance, 199-201
Acid-citrate-dextrose anticoagulation, 74
Actinomyces israelii, 100
Actinomyces naeslundii, 100
Acute glomerulonephritis, 95
Acute lymphocytic leukemia, 35
Acute myelogenous leukemia, 32
Acute myelomonocytic leukemia, 34
Addis count, 82
Addison's disease, 193
Adrenal medulla, 182
Adrenocortical hyperfunction, 178
Adrenocorticotropic hormone, 30, 151, 176-177
Adrenogenital syndrome, 178, 181
Affinity, 119
African sleeping sickness, 114
Agglutination, 44
Agranulocytosis, 28
AHG; *see* Antihemophilic globulin (factor VIII)

t indicates reference to table.

Air
  alveolar, 201
  atmospheric, 201
Air embolism, 73
Air segmentation, 139
Alanine transaminase, 155
Albumin, 150
Alder-Reilley anomaly, 40
Aldolase, 170
Aleukemic leukemia, 36
Alkaline phosphatase
  in adults, 163
  in infants, 163
  stability of, 164
Alkaline phosphatase isoenzyme, 160
Allergen, 22
Alpha particle, 84
Alpha$_1$-antitrypsin, 127
Alpha-1-globulins, 150
Alpha-2-globulins, 150
Alphanumeric language, 142
Amniocentesis, 69-70
Amorph, 50
Amphotericin B, 97
Amylase
  and abdominal pain, 166
  urinary, 167
Amylase isoenzymes, 165
Anaerobic cultures, 99
Analog information, 141
Anamnestic response, 119
Anaphylatoxin, 119
Anaphylaxis, 73
Androgen, production of, 174
Anemia(s)
  aplastic, 4, 18, 90
  causes, 12
  defined, 12

211

White blood cells
   formation site, 20
   function, 21-22
   life span, 21-22
   types, 20
White blood count values, 23-24
Whooping cough, 27
Widal test, 125
Window, 87
Wood's light, 116
Wright's stain, 100, 114

X

Xg blood group system, 59, 61
X-rays, 85

Y

Yeasts, 116
Yersinia enterocolitica, 96

Z

Zimmermann reaction, 175